THE HOMOEOPATHIC TREATMENT OF ALCOHOLISM

By
DOCTOR GALLAVARDIN

GYAN

Published by

GYAN

Gyan Publishing House
5, Ansari Road
Daryaganj, New Delhi-110002
Phone: 011-47034999, 9811692060
E-mail: books@gyanbooks.com

Distribution Network
gyanbooks.com
India, USA, Canada, UK, Australia, France

ISBN : 978-81-212-6603-1 (PB)
First Published, 1890

2nd Impression 2022

Printed at: Gyan Press, Delhi.

THE HOMOEOPATHIC TREATMENT OF ALCOHOLISM
Author: DOCTOR GALLAVARDIN

THE HOMOEOPATHIC TREATMENT OF ALCOHOLISM

THE
Homœopathic Treatment
OF
Alcoholism.

BY

DOCTOR GALLAVARDIN,

OF LYONS, FRANCE.

TRANSLATED FROM THE FRENCH BY

IRENÆUS D. FOULON, A.M., M.D., LL.B.,

Professor of Medical Jurisprudence in the Homœopathic Medical College of Missouri; Managing Editor of the "Clinical Reporter," etc., etc.

1890.

PREFATORY NOTE.

UNDER the title of "The Homœopathic Treatment of Alcoholism," there is here offered to the homœopathists of the United States a translation of the essential portions of Dr. Gallavardin's recent work, entitled "*Alcoholisme et Criminalité. Traitement Médical de l'Ivrognerie et de l'Ivresse.*" The portions of the original work omitted in this translation treat of the evils of intemperance in the use of alcoholic beverages, the work of "temperance" societies in the United States, and the harmful results of limiting the teaching of medical science to institutions under State control—interesting questions, interestingly discussed by the author, but not at all vitally connected with the practical and therapeutic portions of his work. The latter are given entire.

Dr. Gallavardin's monograph is (the translator believes) the first ever written from the homœopathic standpoint upon the important subject of which it treats; it therefore fills, or at least occupies, a void that has hitherto existed in the literature of homœopathy. While the translator wishes it distinctly understood that he in no wise stands sponsor for Dr. Gallavardin's statements, he believes that the author's acknowledged ability and the international reputation he has earned by long years of study, experience and literary labors, as well as the intrinsic importance of the subject, whether viewed from the standpoint of therapeutics, economics or morals, should and will command the respectful attention and study of all thoughtful homœopathists.

Skepticism is either the life or the death of scientific progress. When it is joined to an active love of truth and leads to investigation, it is an element of growth; but when, as is too often the case in the mentally indolent, it degenerates into blind prejudice and dogmatic denial without examination, it becomes a remediless blight upon all intellectual advancement. As the author well states in the body of the work, experiment is the only true test in the experimental sciences. Experiment is all he asks for his system, and, surely, less than that should not be granted. If this translation shall lead any considerable number of thoughtful, honest men to try the author's methods, to the end that they may be either confirmed or disproved, the establishment of the truth, whatever it may be, will be sufficient reward for

THE TRANSLATOR.

Treatment of Alcoholism.

I.

A FEW drunkards can be cured by means of moral instruction, care in diet and hygiene, but, in the far larger number, the tendency to inebriety is the result of a species of morbid impulse which is well-nigh irresistible. This is admitted by Dr. Monin, who, in his work on Alcoholism, says that "the desire for drink is a kind of mental perversion *beyond the rational resources of morals and medicine.* This representative of allopathic medicine declares that, generally, both ethics and medicine are unable to cure drunkenness.

Hitherto homœopathic medicine has proved itself quite as unable to cure drunkenness, because, with rare exceptions, homœopathic physicians, not knowing how to utilize the wealth of their materia medica, have failed to follow these two precepts of their master, Hahnemann:

1st. In the choice of remedies, note the intellectual and moral symptoms presented by the patient and produced by the drug proved upon the healthy subject.

2d. In chronic diseases, give in one dose the remedy selected, then let it act for weeks and months.

Having followed, on these two points, the precepts of Hahnemann, I have been able to cure inebriates of their vice in one-half of my cases, when the vice was not hereditary, and that by causing to be administered to them, without their knowledge, in their food or their drink, the remedy selected for each of them. Further on I shall give the differential indications of fourteen remedies which clinical experience has proved to be efficacious against inebriety, and which may assist other means in curing men of this vice.

I earnestly advise those physicians who have taste and aptitude for this branch of therapeutics to endeavor to complete, by their own experiments, my clinical studies of this subject. They may be able to discover what I have failed to grasp, and, in that way, extend the field of this new therapeutics. As for the physicians who have neither taste nor aptitude for it, let them let it alone, lest they should compromise it by their lack of success. *Natura repugnante, omnia vana*, says Hippocrates, very justly.

Physicians have hitherto practiced only a species of veterinary medicine applied to man, since they have treated in him only somatic or bodily symptoms, and seldom, or at least not daily, psychical symptoms.

From 1854 until 1874 I practiced, like other physicians, this species of veterinary medicine on man. But, since 1871, results, at first rare, then more and more numerous, observed among my patients, have demonstrated to me that it is possible to practice on man a really human medicine, by curing him not only of his diseases, but also of his passions and failings. My conviction on this point has grown little by little, at the same time as my experimental knowledge in the treatment of psychical symptoms. When I had so far progressed as to be able, as I thought, to apply this psychical treatment, I was not satisfied to give the benefit of my knowledge to a few persons among my paying *clientèle*, who were being treated for divers ailments, but determined to give the poor the benefit of this treatment, and, to that end, opened on February 6th, 1886, a free dispensary for psychical treatment, which has been continued since then every Tuesday morning. From twelve to thirty-six persons are to be seen there every Tuesday, seeking for some member of their families this moralizing treatment, as yet unknown to academies and scientific societies!

There are, in all, six means of moral and intellectual culture, three of which are immaterial—religion, education, instruction—and three are material—medication, diet, climate. In another work, as yet unpublished, I have examined how one can use these six means of moral culture, sometimes simultaneously, sometimes alternately, sometimes alone. Here I shall speak only of those remedies whose properties have been studied experimentally, according to the homœopathic law. In this matter I have been preceded by Hahnemann, Hering, Count de Bonneval (of Bordeaux), Canon de Cesoles (of Nice), Bourgeois (of Roubaix), Charles Dulac (of Paris), and Valiaux. If, on this topic, I have been able to gather more data than most of them, it is because I have come last, endeavoring to complete the work they have begun, and because I was the first to establish a dispensary for psychical treatment—an unfailing source of instruction. During the first thirty-four months of the establishment of this dispensary I gave 2,155 consultations—1,431 for drunkards and 725 for libertines and persons suffering from jealousy, envy, irascibility, avarice, laziness, etc., etc.

Unless they be inconsistent, homœopathic physicians must conform their practice to the teachings of Hahnemann (Organon, §210-230) and treat both somatic and psychical symptoms, and the psychical symptoms alone when they exist alone, as the manifestation of a latent morbid condition or of the individual disposition.

The knowledge of psychical effects may even aid legal medicine, as the following fact demonstrates: In 1865, while I was in Münster attending Bœnninghausen's clinic, he said to me one day: "While on a trip in my official capacity as *Regierungsrath*, I met in a hotel certain magistrates who were about to begin an inquest concerning the alleged poisoning, by means of arsenic, of a husband by his wife. 'If you will tell me the moral and intellectual symptoms felt by that man just before his death, I shall probably be able to tell you whether arsenic was the poison used and whether any of it will be found in the stomach of the deceased. Did he, before dying, manifest frightful despair or great serenity?' 'Very great despair,' replied the magistrates. 'Then,' said I, 'he was poisoned by arsenic in so large a dose that some of it will be found in the digestive tract. This drug produces a terrible despair through its primary effect, and perfect serenity through its secondary effect, when the organism is able to react against the primary effect.' There was arsenic found, at the autopsy, in the viscera of that man. In the neighborhood of Münster," adds Bœnninghausen, "a woman poisoned sixteen persons with arsenical omelets. If the allopathic physicians had known the psychical effects of that substance, they would have discovered the poisoning before that woman had caused the death of so many persons."

In applying treatment to passions, I do nothing new. Hahnemann did it before me, and I am only following his scientific method and the tradition of psychical treatment, which can be traced into the night of ages, for at all times and everywhere men have used drugs to re-establish the very unstable equilibrium of their moral and intellectual state.

Diodorus Siculus, the historian, speaks of a drug used by the Egyptians which they called "The antidote to anger and sorrow." This drug contained ***datura stramonium***, which, according to homœopathic physicians, alleviates anger and sorrow.

In the Odyssey, IV. 220, Homer says, "Forthwith, Helen throws into the wine which Telemachus was drinking the drug which drives away sorrow, dissipates anger and causes all ills to be forgotten."

Hippocrates prescribed mandragora against sadness leading to suicide.

According to Aulius Gellius and Valerius Maximus, the Athenian orators, envious of true glory, took, following the example of Carneades, and to strengthen their brain, a dose of hellebore before speaking. Now, according to homœopathic teaching, this remedy develops the memory and the faculty for improvisation.

Among the plants surrounding an old

chateau, those that belong to the war-like epochs of the Middle Ages are excitants, tonics, etc.; the rest, plants of the *Renaissance* period, are aphrodisiacs and depuratives. Thus men are seen having recourse, according to epochs, to divers drugs to assist their favorite passion.

According to a proverb of the Chinese, who have been using that beverage for centuries: "Tea makes the soul placid and calm, and the sight clear and piercing."

Wine was employed by the ancients, as it is by the moderns, as a psychical remedy.

"Wine rejoices the heart of man," says the Bible.

"Wine," writes Galen, "manifestly dissipates all species of sorrow and discouragement, for every day we take wine to that end."

In the second book *De Legibus*, Plato recommends wine "as a preventive of the peevishness of old age, wine which scatters pain and moroseness, wine which softens the hardness of the soul and makes it easier to fashion, like unto fire, which softens iron."

"Wine makes one eloquent," says Aristotle, and it has been used for that purpose by writers (*e.g.*, J. P. Richter, Maimbourg), by composers (*e.g.*, Handel) and by many orators.

"Is there a drinker," says Horace, "whom wine has not made eloquent, or an unfortunate whom wine has not freed from his sorrows?"

"*Foecundi calices, quem non fecere Disertum?*"

"*Contracta quem non in Paupertate solutum?*"

—*Lib. I. Ep. V.*

Almost immediately after the ingestion of a moderate quantity of wine, man appears animated, his eyes glitter, he is disposed to be gay, benevolent, demonstratively affectionate. He discovers with candor and without dissimulation his habits, his disposition; whence the adage: *In vino veritas.* Hence, wine is considered as a sort of sociable drink, which can set in unison hearts and minds at a banquet or other festivity.

All shrewd people, from the sly peasant to the diplomat, know how to make use of the psychical properties of wine to dissipate momentarily the defects in disposition which may clash with their personal interests.

Mark, for instance, at some fair, a peasant buying a milk cow! In order to find out exactly the quality and quantity of milk given by this cow, he will endeavor to modify to his own advantage the disposition of the seller. The latter may be a deceiver, a liar, a thief, or merely exorbitant in his price. The buyer, in order to temporarily dissipate these failings, which are prejudicial to his interests, drags the seller to the public house, treats him to a few glasses of wine, and, little by little, this beverage induces the seller to tell all he did not mean to tell, to do what he did not mean to do. In such a case, wine may sometimes develop good natural impulses.

While, in order to accomplish his purpose, the peasant in the pot-house makes use of the common local wine, the diplomat, in his sumptuous dining-room, offers choice wines, foamy champagne. Diplomat and peasant alike, however, subject their guests to a sort of psychical treatment, and that quite unconsciously, just as Molière's "Mr. Jourdan" wrote prose without knowing it.

According to the size of the dose, wine produces divers, nay opposite, effects. In small doses, it cheers, it revives all the faculties of the soul, it rests and comforts the wearied mind as well as the tired body; but used in excess, it gives a false courage, makes one indiscreet, quarrelsome, aggressive, angry, and leads to a low tone of intellect and morals and to suicide.

Drunkenness transforms an active, laborious, neat man into an apathetic, lazy, unclean, filthy fellow. It provokes impulses to libertinism, jealousy, anger, hatred, suicide and homicide under hallucinations.

The thirty-five kinds of alcoholic drinks consumed by the different nations of the world produce very different psychical effects.

For instance, beer leads to dullness of mind as well as heaviness of body, to a departure from elevated and delicate sentiments to groveling desires.

Cider and pear-cider produce nearly the same effects as beer.

Absinthe, even in small doses, makes one essentially ill-natured and quarrelsome.

Brandy makes the drinker angry and aggressive.

Anisette (*Kümmel*) in small doses clears the brain.

Cherry-brandy (*Kirschwasser*) acts like *anisette*.

Ebriety manifests itself by psychical symptoms which are as varied as the alcoholic drinks which produce them. For instance, alcohol produced from potatoes and grain [owing to the presence of a variable amount of amyl alcohol, otherwise "fusel oil."—*Translator*] produces a comatose ebriety, while alcohol made from wine [pure ethylic alcohol.—*Tr.*] produces a merry, noisy or angry ebriety.

In order to convince the reader that the use of the psychical treatment is as general as it is unconscious, I will quote from professors, physicians, who although ignorant of the name and existence of the psychical treatment, show us that it is daily practiced by millions of men. Two of these professors will describe, the one as a social, the other as an intellectual drink, the infusion of tea-leaves, which numbers from five to six hundred millions of consumers.

"The action of tea," writes Prof. Marvaud, of the Val de Grace, "manifests itself by an agreeable stimulation, accompanied by a feeling of comfort. The individual feels happy at being alive, the faculties of the mind blossom forth, and a mild and pleasant quietude takes possession of our being. Everything seems smiling here below; we love our hosts or our guests better; we readily forgive the shortcomings of our fellows and as readily forget our own faults. We remain silent and lose the consciousness of our misfortunes and annoyances, past and present."

"Tea," writes Prof. Moleschott, of Turin, "increases the power to note impressions received. It disposes one to pensive meditation; and, notwithstanding an increased rapidity in the movement of ideas, the attention is more easily concentrated upon a determinate object. One experiences a feeling of comfort and gayety. The creative activity of the brain maintains itself within the limits imposed to the attention, instead of wandering in pursuit of ideas foreign to the subject-matter under consideration. Seated about the tea-table, men are inclined to keep up a well-ordered conversation, to go to the root of questions under discussion; and the calm gayety which tea produces usually leads them to satisfactory results."

"Tea," says Dr. Monin, "gives wings to

the mind, and to the intellect finish and airiness of inspiration."

But these pleasant moral or intellectual effects are primary effects, lasting a few hours at most, and they are followed by the secondary effects of tea, which are baneful and persistent. Dr. Dulac was, therefore, quite right when he wrote to me: "Through its secondary effect, tea makes one indifferent; and, in the course of time, selfish; tea makes one lonesome and dissatisfied (*ennuyé*), and gradually leads to melancholia." International pride and melancholia are notoriously characteristic of the two nations of Europe and Asia who consume the greatest amount of tea.

Dr. Monin also considers tea as one of the causes of melancholia, and Fothergill attributes to it the constantly increasing nervousness of the youth.

"The name of 'intellectual drink,' which has been given to coffee, indicates clearly its cephalic and exhilarating action," writes Prof. Fonssagrives, of Montpelier. "There is no one who has not noted upon himself, and with sensual satisfaction, the effects which this drink produces. The brain is gently stimulated, it escapes, in a degree, the heavy realties of life and the yoke of weariness. The senses become keener and work with more precision; the imagination is more lively, work is easier; the combinations of the mind crowd upon each other; less solid, perhaps, they are more rapid, clearer; the memory is unusually active, ideas flow with unwonted ease. The mind throws off disagreeable thoughts, becomes freer and more lively, while, at the same time, a feeling of benevolence spreads over the entire being."

There is, of course, a coffee inebriety which is more distinguished and less dangerous than that produced by alcohol, but which, to a certain extent, also demands the warnings and watch-care of hygiene. Men who labor intellectually are oftener than others the victims of this amiable vice, and if they give themselves up to it thoroughly they fall into a state of nervous erethism and emaciation. When Mme. de Sévigné said, "Coffee makes me stupid," she alluded less to the present influence of coffee than to the state of cerebral inertia which follows its action. I know people whose brain works slowly and with difficulty as long as the spur of coffee is wanting; I know others who cannot forego this beverage without suffering from sick headache. From that point of view, it is an evil, as are all servitudes.

Another question, akin to this and which also pertains to the hygiene of literary people, would be to determine exactly the sum and nature of the assistance which coffee lends to thought. There is a cerebral excitement, undeniably, but all the faculties are not stimulated in the same degree, hence there is a little incoherence in the intellectual combinations emitted under the pressure of coffee. From personal experience, I should say that they have more rapidity than solidity; they are more numerous, but less profound. The thought is less free; it is mastered with difficulty; *the judgment and the will are weakened;* and as for me, I long ago gave up this inconvenient stimulation when I am to speak in public. Let poets continue to sip the beverage "dear to them" (Delisle), but let philosophers and scientific men abstain from it; they will be better off for it.

The use of wine, tea, coffee and other psychical remedies, to render the intellectual faculties more active and developed, is really child's play by the side of what homœopathic treatment can accomplish in that respect. Those who use the drugs I have mentioned above utilize only their primary effects, which last but a few hours and are followed by an intellectual depression equal to the artificially produced excitement. Homœopathic physicians, on the contrary, utilize the secondary effects of their remedies, which, especially when they are administered in very high dilutions, may last weeks, months, years, and sometimes indefinitely. This fact is demonstrated by the following

ILLUSTRATIVE CASE.—A young lady, 20 years of age, had so little gift for spoken or written improvisation that, before writing a letter, she was compelled to make one or two sketches or copies of it. Unbeknown to her, I gave her Pulsatilla 200, indicated by the totality of the symptoms. A few weeks later I heard that she was writing her letters without preliminary outlines or copies. And this effect of the remedy has now lasted two or three years and may continue indefinitely. Compare this result with the action of wine or coffee, which, in speakers, develops the faculty for improvisation during three, four, five or six hours only.

By reproducing in this connection my manuscript chapters upon these novel questions, I could more completely set forth the numerous psychical effects of the thirty-four principal kinds of alcoholic beverages upon their six hundred millions of consumers, of tea upon its five hundred millions of consumers, of tobacco upon its two hundred millions of consumers, of coffee upon its one hundred millions of consumers, of betel upon one hundred millions of Hindoos, of opium upon one hundred millions of Asiatics, of hashish upon several millions of Egyptians and Asiatics, of maté upon fifteen millions of South Americans, of coca upon fifteen millions of South Americans, of arsenic upon thousands of people in Austria and in the United States of America, of the musk-toad-stool upon the Laplanders, of the falezlez upon the negroes; but I think it has been sufficient to note, even incompletely, a few of the psychical effects of wine, tea and coffee to show that men, always and everywhere, have felt the urgent need of having recourse themselves to psychical remedies, since hitherto the physicians have not satisfied this want and have been content, I repeat it, to practice a species of veterinary medicine upon man, treating only his somatic or bodily symptoms.

At the present time the Persians, after a rather severe novitiate, use a drug which seems to procure for them the pleasures of the passion which they prefer. The Egyptians, without a preliminary novitiate, make use of another drug, which seems to procure for them also, in some cases at least, the pleasure of their favorite passion. These facts were reported long ago in French and German medical journals.

The use of these divers psychical drugs is so frequent, the drugs themselves are so numerous, that one could apply the German proverb, "The trees prevent your seeing the forest," to those superficial observers who do not see that this psychical treatment is as widely as it is unconsciously used. The soldiers of the Argentine Republic, who prefer tobacco and maté to food, call these two substances, in their incorrect but picturesque language, "*Los vicios de entretenimiento*" (vices for entertainment). Might not the same name be applied to the numerous psychical remedies in use among all nations?

II.

CERTAIN men, who merely reason and refuse either to observe or experiment, reproach us with violating the freedom of our patients' will when we administer psychical remedies to them. But these are the very men who, by absorbing the eleven psychical substances mentioned above, frequently, if not habitually, weaken their judgment, their freedom, their will, and even their morality, since some of these substances (alcoholics, coffee, maté, coca, arsenic, etc.) are aphrodisiacs. We, on the contrary, by means of psychical treatment, moderate passionate impulses, develop reason, the sense of duty, the will to accomplish it, and consequently the freedom which every man has, in varying degrees, to resist personal or hereditary tendencies to evil.

After having noted above the dangers and counter-indications of alcohol, Mr. de Parville forgot to make known its advantages and indications. These were set forth by Dr. Bayes at the Homœopathic Medical Congress held in Manchester, September 9th, 1875. I will now proceed to condense and complete Dr. Bayes' observations.

The muscular beats of the normal heart represent one-fifth of the total muscular expenditure of the body. Those beats are accelerated by labor, by walking, by ingestion of alcohol.

Let a man at rest, seated or lying down, with, say, sixty heart-beats per minute, drink a glass of strong wine or of brandy, and from fifteen to thirty minutes later the number of his heart-beats will increase to eighty, ninety or a hundred per minute.

In a healthy man at rest you count sixty throbs of the pulse at the wrist per minute. The same man, after one or two hours of marching or working, will have a pulse of eighty, ninety or a hundred per minute.

The muscular expenditure of the heart is, therefore, increased by alcohol as much as by walking. But if alcohol is given to a man immediately before a march of several hours' duration, these two causes—the alcohol and the march—will be seen to doubly accelerate the beating of the heart, and consequently to double the expenditure of the heart's muscular force, whence comes a more rapid and noticeable exhaustion of the strength. Hence, it is noticed that soldiers who indulge in alcoholic drinks before beginning a march tire easily and rapidly, and sometimes are quite unable to keep up with their more abstemious comrades. The latter, however, who partake of alcoholic beverages only when the march is over, are rid of the feeling of weariness, and made to feel strong again by these drinks taken in small quantities. In these cases alcohol acts as a homœopathic remedy, according to the law, "Likes cure likes."

Upon the one hand, alcohol, administered to a man at rest, increases the number of the heart-beats, and hence the heart expenditure; upon the other hand, alcohol, administered, in smaller doses especially, to a man after a march or after labor, diminishes rapidly the number of the heart-beats, and hence the sum of heart expenditures, and removes the feeling of physical weakness. I will now explain why the feeling of lassitude disappears sooner under the influence of alcohol.

If, after several hours of march, which

have caused the pulsations of his heart to increase in number from sixty to one hundred per minute, a man sits or lies down to rest, the muscular expenditure of his limbs will cease immediately; not so the muscular expenditure of the heart, which continues much the same as during the march. It is only little by little that the number of the heart-beats diminishes, falling gradually from 100 to 95, 90, 85, 80, 75, 70, 65 and finally 60 per minute. One, two or three hours have elapsed before this gradual moderation is completed, and during that time the muscular expenditure of the heart constitutes at first one-third, then one-fourth, and finally one-fifth of the total muscular expenditure of the body, which is the normal proportion. But if the soldier, immediately after a long march, takes a swallow of alcoholic liquor, it reduces in from fifteen to forty minutes the beating of the heart, whose muscular expenditure, rapidly diminished, soon returns to its normal amount. At the same time and in the same ratio that the number of the heart-beats diminishes the respiratory movements also diminish. Hence a double diminution in the expenditure of the muscular power of the soldier, whose rest or sleep then more rapidly restores his general strength.

When the acceleration of the heart-beats has been caused, not by labor or marching, but by intense heat, such as that of the torrid zone, for instance, and when this feverish acceleration prevents sleep, with its restorative influence, alcohol in small quantities, drunk in the evening *after sunset*, quickly produces balmy sleep. This was noticed by Stanley in Africa, and later by myself in the South of France.

Observation 1.—Stanley has noted that the use of alcoholic beverages is extremely dangerous, indeed deadly, to the Europeans who sojourn in Central Africa. It produces in them mania, liver complaints and sunstroke, even when they are in their tents. But if they drink it in small quantities, in the evening *after sunset*, the frequency of the heart-beats produced by the intense heat diminishes, and they soon fall into a restful sleep, which permits them to attend to their business on the morrow with undiminished strength and vigor.

Observation 2.—A Lyons merchant, whose

business compelled him to travel during the greatest heat of summer in Languedoc, had noted that the heat prevented his sleeping calmly and restfully. Taught by Stahley's experience, I advised him to take in the evening, *after sunset*, a small drink (15 to 30 grammes) of brandy. This always brought about the desired sleep in his case, as well as in that of a friend of his who used the same means.

OBSERVATION 3.—But, as in such cases the proper dose of alcohol may be overstepped and evil result, it seems to me proper to mention some other remedies which have also the property of dissipating fatigue. These are:

1st. According to Dr. Ozanam, the infusion of *Hieracium pilosella*;

2d. According to Dr. Moore, a few drops of the tincture of *Gelsemium sempervirens*;

3d. According to a botanist, Mr. Boulu, the infusion of the entire plant in bloom of *Asperula odorata*;

4th. The tincture of *Arnica*—a few drops in a glass of water.

5th. Aconite, which diminishes the beating

of the heart and thus lessens the mechanical expenditure of the heart. After each day's march a young soldier easily dissipated his fatigue by drinking at one draught a glass of water, into which he had dropped two drops of Aconite—mother tincture. This would be the most comfortable and advantageous means to adopt, since Aconite cures, and may prevent, the consequences of the chilling which so often occurs after a march.

Again, alcohol is a very efficacious remedy against certain morbid conditions. For instance, brandy and rum may save the life of persons who have been bitten by the most venomous snakes, provided they be drunk after the bite has been inflicted. [The truth of this statement is, to say the least, doubtful. —*Tr.*] Dr. Henry Blanc, ex-prisoner of Emperor Theodoros, has noted that, in the Orient, the best remedies for the intermittents of the hot countries are sulphate of quinine and alcohol, administered in alternation.

III.

IN the books on Homœopathic Therapeutics I find recommended, on the strength of the homœopathic theory, more than forty remedies for drunkenness which may be efficacious if they are indicated by the totality of the somatic and psychical symptoms in the person to be treated. But not being able as yet to make their differential indications thoroughly precise, I will now mention the remedies which, as the result of clinical experience, seem to be the most efficacious. I briefly state their differential indications, which my fellow-physicians will complete by seeking for the remedies best indicated, according to the law *similia similibus curantur* in the person to be treated.

1. **Nux vomica.**—Violent people, often cross, and whom sorrows or cares lead to drink as a means of forgetting, and who spit frequently; or mild-tempered people, kind and affectionate in their ordinary condition, who, while drinking, become brutal even to striking, insulting, sometimes weeping. Tendency to jealousy, to envy, to suicide by

shooting or stabbing, before and during drunkenness. Inclination to sadness, or to great genital excitement during drunkenness. Easily made drunk by a small quantity of alcoholic drink. Longing for red wine, white wine, beer, absinth, rum; persons inclined to get drunk for lack of anything else to do; neurotic men, and women addicted to drunkenness during or after pregnancy. Licentious, but only in imagination; still sometimes really immoral; mania for refusing treatment even in urgent cases. Sometimes thieving and shrewd; inclined to cônstipation, to vomiting, to regurgitations, to difficult digestion. Using tobacco, inclined to gamble, spending their entire wealth little by little. Spending through ostentation; close toward his family, open-handed to strangers, avoiding any society but his own family.

2. **Lachesis.**—Ill-natured people, hard to get along with. Inclined to violent crimes, vindictive, wicked, jealous, envious, licentious. Inclined to kill others, but not to kill themselves, except to get themselves run over by a vehicle. Talking ceaselessly before or during drunkenness. Saying or doing while drunk what they would not say or do before.

Appetite for brandy and absinth. Tobacco users. Sometimes spending too freely, sometimes close-fisted; inconsequential.

3. **Causticum.** — Fussy, quarrelsome, cheating, much inclined to be moved to tears before and after drink; very great genital overexcitement before and during drunkenness. Desire for brandy and wine. Indicated for persons who have lost their loved ones. Adults lacking in common sense. Great indifference. Sometimes inclined to theft. Tobacco users. Unable to stand continence. Young girls burning with the desire of marrying. Spendthrifts.

4. **Sulphur.**—Psoriatics. Sufferers from hemorrhoids. Persons who work and go to sleep slowly with a prolonged but not restful sleep. Slow-going people, getting drunk in secret. Having neither the sentiment of duty nor strength of will to accomplish duty. Desire for wine and whisky. Mild before and brutal during drunkenness. More intelligent while they are drunk; saying and doing while drunk what they would neither say nor do before. Obese and corpulent people. Thoughtless, harum-scarum. Inclined to steal and to lie. Envious, somewhat

licentious. Sometimes shrewd and thieving. Tobacco users, gamblers. At times close-fisted, at others inclined to spend through lack of economy.

5. **Calcarea carbonica.**—Corpulent, obese people. Having neither the sentiment of duty nor the strength of will to accomplish it. Not disposed to be obliging. Having motiveless dislike for certain persons. Inclined to steal and to lie. After excessive mental labors, which have weakened the intellect, and inspire a fear of losing their mind. Envious, hateful, vindictive, somewhat licentious. Sometimes inclined to gamble. At times close in money matters, at others spending quite freely for themselves or for show. Devoid of will-power and unable to refuse a glass of wine.

6. **Hepar sulphuris.**—Persons who are not affectionate, always dissatisfied, high-tempered, easily angered, even to homicide. Inclined to be criminal. Needing wine to be able to work mentally.

7. **Arsenicum album.**—Wicked, vindictive, merciless, sometimes jealous; inclined to commit crimes. Inclined to suicide, by stabbing, poisoning or hanging. Persons who

are always thirsty and take any kind of drink, even water. Inclined to vomiting, and more still to diarrhœa; much inclined to persecute others.

8. **Mercurius vivus.**—Always dissatisfied with everything, everybody, and themselves. Inclined to caries of the teeth, to engorgement of the gums, to salivation, neuralgia, diarrhœa, dysentery, intestinal worms. Great gamblers. Sometimes spending freely and sometimes close-fisted. Spending day by day what they earn. Hard to get along with and weak-minded. Having diseases which have been palliated rather than cured.

9. **Petroleum.**—Drunkards without energy, without strength of will, unable to refuse a glass of wine, vomiting after the least excess in drink, talking much when they are drunk.

10. **Opium.**—Especially brandy-drinkers. Getting drunk over humiliations, inclined to weep easily. Very gay or stupid or sleepy while drunk. This remedy suits, in the first case, those who get drunk on wine; in the latter, those who get drunk on cider, beer, ethylic or amylic alcohol.

11. **Staphisagria.**—Suits drunkards who

have made an abuse of venereal pleasures. Being unnerved, they imagine they can restore their poor organism by the abuse of alcoholic liquors, rather by means of mild than strong liquors. Sad before, during and after drunkenness. Hypochondriac. Inclined to persecute. Bachelors and, more still, licentious husbands. Onanism. Jealous. Tobacco users.

12. **Conium maculatum.**—People who drink to "brace up," because they feel extremely lonesome, cold and chilly. Persons who cannot stand continence. Great indifference. Intelligence not as yet thoroughly developed. Adults lacking in reason, like children. Paralytic weakness of the lower spine, and especially of the lower legs, inclined to paraplegia.

13. **Pulsatilla.** — People who imagine they strengthen their stomachs by drinking, and whose digestive powers are really insufficient. Sad while they are drunk. Desire for cider. Chlorotic women and girls who drink for the purpose of gaining strength. Jealous, and still more envious, inclined to hate. Spendthrifts through ostentation. Timid, and even cowardly.

14. **Magnesia carbonica.**—Suits drinkers of mild liquors, those who make very frequent use of dainties and candies. Shrewd, sad, taciturn or loquacious. Face livid or scarlet. Sleeplessness during the night. Sleep during the day. Speaking ceaselessly while drunk.

Here are fourteen principal remedies, which, administered in high potencies (200th and above), one single dose for two, three, four, six or seven weeks, partially or completely destroys the inclination to get drunk, and often prevents the manifestations of divers symptoms which are cured during drunkenness—symptoms which I have indicated for each of these remedies.

IV.

I SHALL now mention nine remedies which are indicated for divers symptoms which appear during drunkenness. They are: *Bellad.*, *Canthar.*, *China*, *Coffea*, *Hyosc.*, *Ignat.*, *Phosphor.*, *Stramon.*, *Veratr.* These remedies will generally suffice to dissipate all unpleasant or dangerous symptoms of drunkenness, but then they must be administered in the 3d, 6th, 12th or 30th dilution, six or eight globules dissolved in a half glass of fresh water, and a teaspoonful of this dilution is administered every five, ten, fifteen or twenty minutes. I will mention one example as showing how rapid, at times, is the curative action of the remedy indicated in each case.

CONVULSIVE FORM OF DRUNKENNESS, CURED BY *Nux vom.* Being temporarily in the country, I was called upon to attend a robust young man of 20, who had been made drunk with wine and brandy. His limbs were agitated. His convulsive movements could hardly be restrained by four strong men, who endeavored to hold this young drunkard down upon a bed. I dissolved six or seven globules of *Nux vom.*[30] in a half-glassful of water, and every five minutes I administered a teaspoonful of this solution to the drunk man. After the third spoonful the convulsions disappeared entirely, and the young man became calm and was able to go to sleep, *as is proper in such cases.*

I shall now state the divers symptoms which manifest themselves during drunkenness, and the remedies indicated to cure them.

Convulsive form of drunkenness, with violent contortions of the limbs, of the body, of the head: *Nux vom.*, *Bellad.*

Jealousy: *Nux vom.*, *Laches.*, *Pulsat.*, *Staphis.*, and especially *Hyosc. nig.*

Fury for striking: *Nux vom.*, *Hepar*, *Veratr. alb.*, *Hyosc.*

Fury for destroying everything: *Veratr.*, *Bellad.*

Fury for killing others: *Bellad.*, *Hepar*, *Hyosc.*

Inclination to commit suicide: *Arsen.* (by poisoning, stabbing, hanging, or getting himself run over by a vehicle); *Nux vom.* (by stabbing, firearms or drowning); *Bellad.* (by poisoning, stabbing, hanging, and especially by throwing himself headlong from a high place).

Great gayety: *Opium*, *Coffea.*

Playing comedy: *Stramon.*, *Bellad.*

More intelligent: *Sulphur*, *Calc. carb.*

Stupid: *Opium*, *Stramon.*

Sleepy: *Opium*, *Bellad.*

Impossibility to go to sleep: *Nux vom.*, *Coffea.*

Speaking ceaselessly: *Laches.*, *Caustic.*, *Hepar*, *Petrol.*, *Magn. carb.*

Yelling, shouting: *Stramon.*, *Hyosc.*, *Ignat.*, *Causticum.*

Insulting: *Nux vom.*, *Hepar*, *Petrol.*

Complaining, dissatisfied: before, during and after drunkenness: *Hydrastis canad.*, *Nux vom.*, *Causticum*, *Laches.*

Inclined to strip entirely naked: *Hyosc.*

Great genital excitement: *Nux vom.*, *China*, *Phosphor.*, *Canthar.*, and especially *Causticum.*

Saying what they did not mean to do or say before being drunk: *Laches.*, *Bellad.*, *Sulphur.*

Among the people whom I treated for the cure of drunkenness there are those whose drunkenness continues or is repeated during three, five or eight days in succession. This prolonged drunkenness may have dangerous consequences, both for the drunkards and for those who are about them. For instance, a coachman may fall from his seat or tip over his carriage with the travelers whom it contains. In such cases I give to the relatives or friends of those drunkards *Bellad.*, 12th dilution, and especially *Nux vom.* The relatives dissolve three or four globules of a single remedy in a half-glassful of water, and give a small teaspoonful of this dilution to the drunk persons every five, ten, fifteen or twenty minutes, according as they desire to act more or less promptly. The remedy is given alone or mixed in coffee, wine or tea.

As there are in France (this is equally true of the United States.—*Tr.*) homœopathic pharmacies in only ten or fifteen cities, and allopathic pharmacies in all towns, and even in many villages, I have indicated the remedies which cure drunkenness and which may be procured from allopathic pharmacies, and which are to be administered to drinking persons presenting the following symptoms:

Convulsive movements of the limbs: *Nux vom.*

Fury for destroying everything: *Bellad.*

Fury for striking: *Nux vom.*

Fury for killing others: *Bellad.*

Fury for suicide: *Nux vom., Bellad.*

Insulting: *Nux vom.*

Yelling, shouting: *Stramon., Hyosc.*

Unable to go to sleep: *Nux vom., raw coffee.*

Stupid or sleepy: *Opium, Bellad.*

Inclination to strip naked: *Hyosc.*

Great genital excitement: *Nux vom., Canthar.*

Jealousy: *Nux vom., Hyosc.*

Jealous to the point of killing: *Hyosc.*

Saying and doing what they would not have said or done before being drunk: *Bellad., Sulphur.*

Vomiting: *Nux vom.*

Vomiting, diarrhœa: *Arsenious acid* (solution 1.1000).

It will be sufficient to take a drop of the alcoholic or mother tincture indicated, and to pour this drop into a half-glassful of water, of which a small teaspoonful will be given to the drunk man every five, ten, fifteen or thirty minutes. This will rapidly cure his drunkenness.

Many families, all saloon and innkeepers should procure these remedies to administer to those who might need them, for the benefit of both the drunkards and those about them. There are, I repeat it, two kinds of drunkenness, which are quite different as to treatment. First, acquired drunkenness, which is the easier to cure by means of a few remedies clearly indicated in each individual case. Secondly, hereditary drunkenness, coming from parents who have procreated while in a state of drunkenness, or in whom drunkenness has become a confirmed, habitual vice. In order to cure or prevent the development of hereditary drunkenness, it is necessary to treat the young man, or even the child, before the tendency to drunkenness has manifested itself, by administering to him, for two or three years or more, the thirteen remedies mentioned below, in the following order:

1. *Sulphur.*
2. *Nux vom.*
3. *Arsen.*
4. *Merc. viv.*
5. *Opium.*
6. *Laches.*
7. *Pulsat.*
8. *Petrol.*
9. *Conium.*
10. *Caustic.*
11. *Magn. carb.*
12. *Staphis.*
13. *Calc. carb.*

Each of these thirteen remedies is to be administered in a single dose and in the 200th dilution to the young man, beginning at the age of thirteen or fourteen years. The remedies must be permitted to act for the following length of time:

1. *Sulphur*, . . . forty days.
2. *Nux vom.*, . " "
3. *Arsen.*, . . " "

4.	*Mercur.*,	forty days.
5.	*Opium*,	" "
6.	*Laches.*,	" "
7.	*Pulsat.*,	" "
8.	*Petrol.*,	sixty days.
9.	*Conium*,	" "
10.	*Caustic.*,	" "
11.	*Magn. carb.*,	" "
12.	*Staphis.*,	forty days.
13.	*Calc. carb.*,	sixty days.

To the children of drunkards, who are less than thirteen or fourteen years of age and who are very sensitive to the action of these drugs, the thirteen remedies mentioned above are to be administered in the same order, successively, but only in the 30th dilution. As this dilution has a less protracted action, each remedy is permitted to act only one-half of the time assigned for the same remedy in the 200th dilution. For instance, *Sulphur* during twenty days, *Petrol.* during thirty days, etc.

But when the families of these children, predestined to drunkenness, shall be in frequent communication with a homœopathic physician, the latter will not always administer the thirteen remedies mentioned in the order which I have recommended. He will preferably prescribe, out of the thirteen remedies (and also *Hepar* and others), the one which may be best indicated for each patient by the totality of the somatic and psychical symptoms, which are often violent and numerous in the children of drunkards. By acting thus, the physician will, little by little, cure a patient of his passions and shortcomings, and will, sooner and more easily, prevent the development of hereditary drunkenness. Carried on in this way, the preventive treatment of drunkenness will bring about the somatic and psychical improvement of each youth, upon whom the remedy will really play the part of a means of moral and intellectual culture. Hence it will sometimes occur that the children of drunken parents will, in this way, obtain a more precocious and complete moral and intellectual development than other children. This will, little by little, cause the parents of the latter to give them also the benefit of psychical treatment.

* * * * * *

V.

After having read the differential indications of the remedies which are curative of drunkenness, many readers may believe that they will be able to make, in a short time, numerous cures of this sort. Let them undeceive themselves, for whether through lack of sufficient information in reference to the drunkard, or because of the incomplete knowledge of the properties of the remedies, the choice of the latter is often difficult. I might call as witnesses to this fact the two amiable physicians who, alternately, have the kindness to act as my secretaries, to note the symptoms of the drunkards treated in my dispensary, in order to permit me to attend to a larger number of patients in a given time.

I am often asked how long a time it would take me to cure a given drunkard. I answer that I do not know at all. Among drunkards there are no two who are alike in personal appearance, in temperament, in disposition, in sensitiveness to the action of remedies. Since each of them lives, thinks, acts in his own way, each of them must always be treated in his own manner, which is not that of the others. It is especially in psychical treatment that the physician must govern his conduct according to those two judicious thoughts of Hufeland: "In order that a treatment may be good, it is necessary that a physician should have not copied or imitated, but invented it anew," for "Great talent consists in generalizing diseases and individualizing patients as much as possible." Hahnemann teaches likewise that to each patient there must be administered that remedy which has produced, in a healthy man, the totality of the somatic and psychical symptoms exhibited by the person to be treated.

This individual rule must precede all other rules given by science, by setting forth the differential indications of the divers remedies for drunkenness. In a word, to the physician, art should hold a higher place than science.

These facts furnish us with a glimpse of the treatment of drunkenness and other passions.

VI.

THERE will be noted in the effects of remedies upon drunkards numerous individual diversities, even a few that are contradictory. For instance, under the influence of *Nux vom.* 200th, one drunkard who was made drunk by a glass of wine will be able to drink several glasses without getting drunk at all; another patient, who could not be made drunk with less than two bottles of wine, will thenceforth be made drunk by a single glass of the same wine, which he no longer will be able to stand.

After having taken this remedy unbeknown to himself, one drunkard will no longer have that thirst which leads him to drink wine; another will feel such a repulsion for that drink that he will no longer wish to drink anything but water; a third one, ceasing to be a drunkard, will not change any in disposition; a fourth one, on the contrary, after having been cured of drunkenness, will no longer be jealous, or sensitive, or easily angered, but will become amiable and obliging toward his wife and children. All that precedes gives a glimpse of the numerous individual modifications of dispositions which occur daily under the influence, either of the abandonment of drink, or the action of the remedies administered.

I cannot detail here the observations, daily increasing in number, of men and women of all classes whom I have treated for drunkenness. In order to show the reader what psychical treatment can do against these passions, I shall only mention cases in which drunkenness was cured, rapidly or gradually, by one, two or more remedies; other cases in which drunkenness (ameliorated, or done away with temporarily) again seized its victim, to be again cured by the second treatment, or not to be cured again at all if treatment was not resumed.

OBSERVATION 1.—A young woman, 28 years old, had, for the past six years, been getting drunk on brandy, to such an extent that her husband intended to apply for a divorce. She had formed this vicious habit during her first pregnancy, and, since then, had continued it uninterruptedly. I gave six or seven globules of *Nux vom.* 200th, which were to be dissolved in a third of a glassful of water for a quarter of an hour; then this mixture, after having been thoroughly stirred with a small spoon for eight or ten minutes, was to be poured into a soup, which was also to be thoroughly stirred with a spoon. This soup was to be eaten as the sole article of food for that meal, and no other food or drink was to be taken immediately before or after this. The solution of the remedy can also be poured into a cup of milk, cocoa, chocolate, coffee or tea, into a glass of pure or sweetened water, even into a glassful of wine, or a liquor-glassful of brandy.

This single remedy, which I directed should be thus administered to this lady unknown to her, cured her completely of her drunkenness.

Many readers will perhaps be astonished that a remedy in the 200th or 10,000th dilution, thus administered in food or drink, should nevertheless manifest its remedial properties. Experiments will prove the exactness of the fact, and, what is more, that the diluted remedies, which have passed the point of chemical reaction (as has been shown by Dr. L. L. Lembert), remain unaltered and retain their curative action, even when they are administered in the midst or at the end of a hearty meal. I have noticed this in patients who, having misunderstood my directions, had taken their medicine under these conditions, one of them, for instance, in a cup of coffee just after a meal. In this case a young man, 29 years of age, a former soldier, to whom *Staphis.* 10,000th, had been administered without his knowledge, at intervals of eight months, produced exactly the same effect, which was undeniable in both instances. Still, I avoid, as much as possible, having the remedy taken in this manner.

OBSERVATION 2.—A woman came to my dispensary, saying: "My husband has left me, and I have only my personal labor as a means to provide for my two children; but, unfortunately, I am addicted to a passion which may prevent my accomplishing it. As I keep a small saloon, I am induced unintentionally to drink too much wine and liquor. Have you remedies which would produce in me a disgust for drink?" I placed upon her tongue six or seven globules of *Nux vom.* 200th. Three weeks later she returned, saying: "I no longer have a taste for alcoholic drugs." Two or three weeks later she returned again, saying she was again forming a liking for these drinks. I again administered *Nux vom.* 600th to cure this slight relapse.

OBSERVATION 3.—A married man, aged 39 years, had for ten months been drunk, licentious, very irascible, quarrelsome and loud-mouthed.

February 23d, 1886, he takes, unknown to himself, a dose of *Laches.* 200th.

March 16th, slight amelioration of all his faults.

April 6th, less cross, less irascible, but still drinks. He takes *Laches.* 200th.

May 4th, great amelioration of his disposition, but still drinks a little.

June 2d, he has not been drunk for two weeks and comes home earlier at night.

February 15th, 1887, disposition very kindly, but still drinks a little. He takes *Laches.* 200th.

March 15th, he no longer gets drunk; he is no longer licentious.

April 12th, amelioration continues.

May 24th, the same.

His wife and children have left him and gone he knows not where, but he has not relapsed into drunkenness or licentiousness, two vices which have been cured by a single remedy, taken in three doses, at divers intervals.

OBSERVATION 4.—Consulted by a drunkard, I administered to him one dose of *Nux vom.* 200th or *Laches.* 200th. One year later I learned that he had been so thoroughly cured of his passion that he no longer drank anything but sweetened water, and he felt such a disgust for wine that he had even stopped going to the public house in order to avoid seeing it drunk.

OBSERVATION 5.—A woman, the owner of a vineyard, during her first pregnancy felt a disgust for all food except cheese, on which she fed almost exclusively. As this was insufficient as food, she drank wine in order to keep up her strength, or ate bread dipped in wine. Although she did not like wine, she formed a habit of drinking more and more of it, until she had been getting drunk daily for at least eighteen months. When she drank she lay down, and thus spent one-half of the day in bed. As she drank in secret, I caused to be administered to her, without her knowledge, on the 11th of May, 1882, in a single dose, six or seven globules of *Sulphur* 5000th. This remedy cured her completely of her desire for drink, but a few weeks later she again took to drink, on account of her sorrow at seeing her crop destroyed by hail. Then, in order to dissipate this sorrow and its consequences, I caused to be administered to her, without her knowledge, on the 14th of June, a single dose of *Nux vom.* 10,000th, which cured her for good of her inclination to drink.

OBSERVATION 6.—In a little work of sixty pages, entitled "How Homœopathic Treatment can Better the Disposition of Man and Develop his Intellect," which was published in 1882 in the "Bulletin of the Homœopathic Medical Society of France," then, later at the end of the second volume on my "Clinical Talks," I related the following observation, which I summarize here because it is rather instructive.

A married man, sneaking, jealous, cross, had, for three years, been getting drunk every day, thirty times a month. He neglected his wife, his children, his business, and had spent in drink all his property.

November 19th, 1879, I had him take, without his knowledge, *Laches.* 2000th in a single dose. On the 17th of December following he was no longer jealous at all, and was beginning to be less sneaking and cross, but he got drunk just as often. Then he was given, without his knowledge, *Laches.* 200th in one dose. On the 28th of January, 1880, his wife informed me that her husband had got drunk only five times during the month instead of thirty. His disposition is still improving, he is better to his family and more careful of his business.

On June 9th I learned that he had got drunk only once since the 28th of January preceding.

On the 20th of October I was told that he had got drunk recently five times; then he was given without his knowledge one dose of *Laches.* 2000th.

On the 20th of December I learned that during the last month he had got drunk almost every day, six or seven times a week. Now he gets drunk on the sly. This latter symptom caused me to give him, without his knowledge, one single dose of *Sulphur* 5000th, which cured him of his desire for drink so thoroughly that, at his meals, he drinks only water like the other members of his family.

OBSERVATION 7.—A married man, aged 41 years, psoriatic, industrious, mild-tempered even while drunk, suffered from hereditary alcoholism and had been getting drunk since the age of 13 years.

February 28th, 1886, he takes *Nux vom.* without success.

March 16th, muscular pains in the calf and the hip. He takes *Sulphur* 300th.

April 13th, cured of muscular pains, but the drunkenness is kept up. He takes *Nux vom.* 200th.

May 4th, he still drinks, but can stand less wine. He takes *Causticum* 200th.

June 2d, he has not got drunk since the 4th of May. His will is weak. He takes *Petrol.* 200th.

July 16th, his will is still weak. He takes *Conium* 600th.

August 31st, his reason having been developed by the preceding remedy, he avoids temptations to drink. Will is not strong. He takes *Calc. carb.* 300th.

September 21st, when he has a chance he drinks more and more. Still he is stronger, but his will power is not great. To cure intercurrent diarrhœa he is given *Ars. alb.* 1x, to be taken three or four times a day during several days.

November 2d, cured of the diarrhœa. He has not got thoroughly drunk for five weeks. He is still fond of wine.

November 30th, the amelioration continues. He takes one dose *Ars. alb.* 300th.

December 28th, has not been drunk for four weeks.

January 18th, 1887, the cure continues.

May 24th, he still likes wine, but no longer gets drunk.

June 21st, he takes *Arsen.* 2000th in order to maintain the cure.

July 19th, he has not got drunk since the 1st of January.

October 18th, he still remains entirely sober, but is still fond of wine. To bring about a distaste for it I give him *Hepar* 200th.

Arsen. 200th and 2000th cured this hereditary drunkenness, a disease whose cure is so difficult to accomplish. He has not got drunk for an entire year.

Observation 8.—A married man, 68 years old, the grandson of a drunkard, the son of an ill-natured mother, has been getting drunk for thirty-four years, principally on absinth. He is weak-minded, easily angered for a short time. Aristotle used to say that wine makes one eloquent. Many public speakers use it on that account. During each spree this drunken fellow talked insultingly for six hours at a stretch; the remedies gradually reduced the length of this drunkard's disagreeable talks to five, four, three, two, one, and even one-half hour, diminishing at the same time the insolent character of that species of eloquence. His wife was particularly interested in the gradual diminution of this talk, for she was compelled to remain by his side so long as he was drunk in order to prevent his insulting the neighbors. This woman came to my dispensary every three or four weeks, for more than twenty months in succession, with rare constancy. This permitted me to cure, or to ameliorate, little by little, this chronic drunkenness, which had been lasting for thirty-four years, and into which he relapses occasionally, but which is less intense than it used to be, and occurs at longer intervals of time. The reader will see how I proceeded in this case.

March 30th, 1886, he takes, without knowing it, one dose of *Laches.* 200th.

April 16th, no result. He takes *Causticum* 200th.

May 11th, no result. He takes *Nux vom.* 200th.

June 2d, no result. He takes *Petrol.* 200th.

June 23d, he talks less insulting while drunk, chatters, yells, insults less, and has greater strength of will. Now he talks only two or three hours while he is drunk. He takes *Petrol.* 3000th.

July 13th, he drinks as much as ever, but he yells and insults less while drunk. *Petrol.* 10,000th.

Great amelioration until the 1st of August, when he got very drunk.

August 3d, he takes *Petrol.* 10,000th.

August 24th, he has not got drunk since the 1st—is more reasonable.

August 5th, he is better, talks less, is less insulting toward his daughter.

November 3d, amelioration continues.

November 23d, he takes *Phosphor.* 200th in one dose, for threatening paralysis of the tongue.

December 14th, amelioration continues.

January 11th, 1887, he has got drunk several times, but speaks less.

February 28th, he gets maudlin drunk. He takes *Causticum* 200th.

March 1st, he is more calm, but defiant and cross. This is perhaps a drug aggravation.

March 21st, still ill-natured, talkative, insolent, inclined to use his knife on himself, his family, his neighbors. He takes *Hepar* 200th.

April 19th, amelioration in all respects. He talks only one hour while drunk.

May 17th, amelioration continues.

June 15, amelioration continues. Still he gets drunk on five successive days. Wine no longer produces muscular excitement, hence his relatives mistakenly imagine that he is less strong than formerly.

July 5th, the amelioration continues.

August 2d, likewise.

August 23d, amelioration is more marked: he reasons better. He talks only one-half hour while drunk.

September 20th, amelioration continues.

October 18th, slight relapse. He takes *Hepar* 200th.

November 2d, relapse. December 6th, better.

January 9th, 1888, unchanged. He takes *Hepar* 3000th.

Since then he has at times relapses which have been dissipated principally by *Petrol.* 10,000th.

Observation 9.—A married man, 60 years of age, the son of a drunken father, a drunkard himself, becoming more so since a number of years, usually mild-mannered, but noisy, turbulent and licentious while he was drunk.

January 9th, 1886, he takes, without knowing it, a single dose of *Laches.* 200th.

March 2d, no result. He takes *Nux vom.* 200th.

March 23d, a slight amelioration, preceded by a slight aggravation. He takes *Nux vom.* 600th.

April 13th, no noticeable amelioration; still, he is less ill-tempered and loud while drunk. He takes *Sulphur* 5000th.

May 4th, he is more mild-mannered, more

calm, has not got drunk for three weeks, he cannot stand wine so well, sleeps better.

May 25th, he has been less nervous for the last six weeks.

June 2d, since the 25th of May he has got drunk twice. He takes *Sulphur* 2000th.

June 29th, he gets drunk just as formerly. He takes *Petrol.* 200th.

September 7th, in the same state as before. He takes *Crotal.* 200th.

September 28th, no result. He takes *Causticum* 200th.

November 9th, no result. He takes *Calc. carb.* 300th.

The wife of this drunkard has no hope of success and gives up the treatment, and this quite mistakenly; for if she had persevered, like the wives of some of the subjects mentioned already, I should very probably have succeeded, little by little, in curing her husband's hereditary drunkenness.

OBSERVATION 10.—A married man, 35 years old, the son of a father who had been a lazy fellow and a drunkard for thirty-five years, became a drunkard himself at the age of 16. He is under-handed, vain, mendacious and steals his wife's money for drink. When he is drunk he beats his wife.

April 13th, 1886, he takes *Nux vom.* 200th.

May 4th, no result. He takes *Nux vom.* 10,000th.

May 25th, he is a little less ill-natured, but drinks just as much. He receives *Laches.* 200th.

June 8th, he is less ill-natured, but drinks more.

July 16th, he refuses to work any longer. He receives *Sulphur* 5000th.

July 27th, he takes *Laches.* 30th, two doses in twenty days.

August 24th, he is ill-natured, selfish, rough, and refuses to work. He takes *Calc. carb.* 300th.

September 21st, no change.

March 22d, 1887, he is better-natured, he still drinks, but he no longer steals his wife's money for drink. This proves that he is less given to drink than before.

The mother of this drunkard gave up the treatment, and this quite mistakenly, for I could here make the same remarks as at the end of the preceding observation.

There are sometimes very prompt and encouraging cures, like the three that follow :

OBSERVATION 11.—A married man was accustomed to drink as high as thirty glasses of absinth. After a single dose of *Causticum* 200th, taken without his knowing it, he felt such a repulsion for absinth, and even for wine, that not only did he not drink any more of it, but he could not even remain in the presence of persons who were drinking the stuff.

OBSERVATIONS 12 AND 13.—There was administered to a man and his son-in-law, who were both great drinkers of absinth, without their knowledge, to the one *Laches.* 200th, and to the other *Nux vom.* 200th, which produced in them such a disgust for this liquor that their respective wives smilingly heard them say to one another, " Don't you find that absinth is not good any more ?" " That is so ; I drank some at so and so's, and it was very bad." " And I drank some in such and such a *cafe* which was good for nothing. We will have to give up drinking absinth, for they do not make any more that is good." " That is what I think also, and I am not going to drink any more absinth;" and the two women continued to smile as they overheard this consoling dialogue.

There are drunkards, fortunately not many, whom I treated almost without success for months and months. I at last discovered that in them the dipsomania was hereditary or symptomatic of a mild form of insanity, which had no other manifestations. Drunkenness is difficult to cure in both of these classes of cases, but especially in the latter, for in the first, that of the hereditary drunkards, a certain number are cured if they are as constant in the treatment as the physician himself.

There is a third class of cases, comprising cases of drunkenness, whether hereditary or not, in which drinking has been kept up for twenty, thirty or forty years, and has impressed upon the organism an inveterate habit which has become a species of second nature. Sometimes an almost ceaseless or often repeated treatment is necessary to cure this sort of drunkenness.

In the fourth class of cases, drunkenness, whether hereditary or not, manifests itself not as being the result of physical appetite or protracted habit, but as that of levity or lack of will power. It is sometimes difficult to act upon these people devoid of mental and moral ballast, who float upon the ocean of life, now driven by the waves of their changing caprices, now by the wills of those who surround them. To this class of people it is necessary to administer the indicated remedies, not only for their intermittent dipsomania, but also and especially for their fantastic disposition* and their lack of will power,† which are the predisposing causes thereof. This class of men is often more difficult to cure than others who are ten times worse drinkers, but who have mental and moral ballast. I might add to the preceding observation many others which are as different among themselves as are drunkards among themselves in their personal appearance, temperament and co-existing somatic and psychical symptoms. All these observations would show that drunkenness, when it is not hereditary, can

---

* Fantastic: *Veratr., China, Ipec.*, Natr. carb. Thoughtless, inconsequential: *Arn., Puls., Sulphur, Agar., Laches.*

†*Calc. carb., Sulphur, Merc. sol., Amm. mur., Bar. carb., Lycop., Petrol., Natr. mur., Silicea.*

be cured in one-half of the cases, on condition that the treatment should be continued with persistency, and even should be repeated after relapses occur.

VII.

After having chosen the remedy best indicated by the somatic and psychical symptoms which the drunkards present, it is generally necessary to give this remedy only in the 200th dilution. This sometimes provokes a slight aggravation for a few days. This aggravation, which is a good sign, is usually followed by a partial or complete cure. But the aggravation should not be too great, nor continue for several weeks as I have noted it, for instance, after one single dose of *Sulphur* 5000th, in a few inebriates, not in all; for then the patient is not always able to react, and the aggravation retards, or even prevents, the cure. When the aggravation manifests itself, the remedy should be permitted to act for three, four, six, eight or twelve weeks, after which partial or complete cure takes place.

It is prudent to administer at first the 200th

dilution, and then the 600th, 1000th, 2000th, 4000th, 6000th, 10,000th, 16,000th.

In order to avoid aggravations, a single dose should be administered at once, for if this dose were to be dissolved in a glass of water and a teaspoonful given once or twice a day for several days in succession, there would be great danger of producing an aggravation of the existing symptoms, and this aggravation would sometimes last for days, weeks and months, and the cure would be retarded.

Between the divers remedies or dilutions administered there should be intervals as variable as the effects produced and the person treated. But, as I do for the patrons of my free dispensary, the physician should receive every three weeks a visit from his consultants, either at his office or at his dispensary. That is the best method of watching the case and directing the most rapid and efficacious treatment.

But this treatment will produce no result unless the efficaciousness of the high dilutions administered shall have been verified by the physician in his daily practice, whether these high dilutions come from the homœopathic pharmacy or from the physician's private medicine case. The high dilutions of the remedies are the indispensable instruments for the cure of drunkenness. Without this instrument there are no cures.

VIII.

To make the treatment of drunkenness and, generally speaking, of psychical diseases as efficacious as possible, the following condition is very useful, and, indeed, I might say, generally indispensable. No reproaches should be addressed to the person under treatment, even though he might deserve them richly, and in conversation no allusion should be made to his vices or failings. Reproaches and allusions sour the temper, while remedies sweeten it by developing reason, the sentiment of duty, and will power sufficient to accomplish it. Thus, for instance, up to date I have cured of their vice all the licentious married men whom I have treated except three, two especially whose wives overwhelmed them with reproaches and snappish innuendoes.

After having noted how indispensable it is,

in order to bring about their cure, not to heap reproaches upon drunkards, I understand why in the numerous colony of insane people at Gheel, Belgium, scattered as boarders among the families of from twelve to fifteen villages in this *canton*, insane people who before had been violent and dangerous in other establishments, because they were restrained and roughly handled, became gentle and inoffensive among the inhabitants of this *canton*, who, under the fortunate religious influences which have been perpetuated among them for eight hundred years, are accustomed to treat with the greatest Christian forbearance these beings, bereaved of their reason, whom they leave in complete freedom, treating them as their own children.

There is another condition which generally favors the efficiency of the treatment of drunkenness and other vices: it is to treat all these patients without their personal knowledge, for some, indeed, take pleasure in these vices and do not wish to be cured of them. Among the others, who know they are being treated for these failings, some desire to assist in their own cure and do so awkwardly. They are sometimes disposed to prevent it by the natural spirit of opposition; others still, anxious concerning the result of the treatment, unconsciously prevent its full effect. When, on the contrary, all these vicious people are treated without their knowledge, there is produced in them a natural evolution toward good under the influence of the remedies, which dissipate a more or less irresistible impulse of the passions, and, I repeat it, develop reason, the feeling of duty and the will power necessary for its accomplishment.

Generally, drinking women consult for themselves or through a third person the physician who can cure them of their passion. As for men, the contrary is generally true, for they take pleasure in the vice and do not wish to be cured of it. Hence it is necessary to treat them without their knowledge in almost every case. Women, therefore, more easily than men, can be made to follow certain rules of hygiene which may diminish or extinguish the taste and thirst for alcoholic drinks. Thus, for instance, in the United States, in the asylums for the treatment of the inebriety of wealthy people, they can be cured of this vice only by compelling them to give up the use of meat altogether. The physicians in these asylums, who make no use of the remedies that can cure drunkenness, are entirely right in depriving the inebriates of meat, for meat increases thirst. If you entirely deprive of meat children and adults, you will see both less thirsty and drinking much less, even in the heat of summer. What I would say concerning the disadvantages of meat applies only to the lean part, for the fat, the marrow of the bones and all fatty matters (oil, butter, cream, milk) diminish both thirst and hunger.

The use of tobacco, whether chewed or smoked, contributes also to the increase of thirst.

But it is clear that it will be impossible to make persons addicted to drink give up altogether the use of meat and tobacco, since one is obliged to treat them almost without their knowledge. It is generally advantageous to limit them to very regular meals, not very hearty ones; for instance, four daily meals, almost equal in quantity. When they are thus fed they are less thirsty, feel stronger, and are less inclined to have recourse to alcoholic drinks, either to quench their thirst or to "brace up."

IX.

After having explained the homœopathic treatment of drunkenness, I think it well to make known another treatment of it, empirical in its nature, used by a homœopathic physician in Mexico, Dr. Ezekiel de Leon, and published in 1883 in the *Bibliotheque Homeopathique*, vol. 15, page 26.

Observation 1.—This physician was consulted by a washerwoman, 41 years of age, who had been addicted for the last twelve years to alcoholic drinks, and already presented the following serious condition: Epistaxis, petechiæ, hemorrhage from the gums and the rectum, convulsions, etc. He had her to take every morning, on an empty stomach, fifty centigrams of tartar emetic in ninety grams of brandy, her favorite liquor. At the end of a few days the patient began to feel such a horror for alcoholic drinks that the very sight of them nauseated her. After the treatment had been suspended for twenty-eight days it was resumed for a few days, after which the cure was complete and permanent. To-day the patient has such a horror of alcohol that she cannot stand the odor of remedies which contain any. She has become industrious, actively attends to her household duties, and presents no longer any signs of her former very grave nervous state.

OBSERVATIONS 2, 3, 4, 5, 6, 7, 8.—Later, Dr. De Leon submitted to the same treatment seven drunkards belonging to different trades. Four were cured, one died because he had reached too advanced a period of alcoholism. In the other two, who suffered from hereditary dipsomania, the result was incomplete.

This emetic treatment, since it does not cure hereditary drunkenness, is inferior to homœopathic medication. Still, when the latter does not act with sufficient speed, one might prescribe emetic dissolved in the alcoholic drinks preferred by the drinker. But in order to avoid all (even slight) poisoning by the emetic, it should be prescribed only in graduated does of five, ten, fifteen, twenty, twenty-five centigrams, and should not be pushed beyond a dose which produces vomiting or diarrhœa in the patient. To children, doses of one, two, three, five, ten centigrams only should be given, but always exclusively in their alcoholic drink, in order to disgust them with it by giving it a nauseous taste.

In England this medication has been at times used in asylums for inebriates. The drink of the latter should be mixed with tartar emetic, which acquires the nauseous taste that inspires the inebriates with a distaste for alcohol, which has sometimes been persistent.

The practice of my dispensary has given me another indication for emetic. This remedy, administered in the morning in a cup of coffee or in soup, brings about a nauseous state of the stomach which continues, and thenceforth takes away from drunkards the desire to drink during that day. The emetic should therefore be administered to them on Saturday, the weekly pay day, or on Sunday, a day of rest, which is devoted to their libations. The emetic, dissolved in a warm vehicle (such as coffee, soup, tea), induces nausea more thoroughly than when not dissolved in a warm vehicle. I have in this manner often prescribed with success tartar emetic to drunkards in whom most remedies had proved inefficacious for months and months. For instance, an inebriate, 68 years of age, who had been getting drunk three, four or five times a week for thirty or forty years, remained sober for three months, during which he only got drunk once, and then but little. He was subject to diarrhœa, which was brought on by emetic in a dose of two and one-half centigrams. There were homœopathic indications for this remedy. It is necessary to try little by little what dose is appropriate to each subject, in order to avoid all poisoning.

In Sweden the inebriates are isolated, and all their meals are seasoned with *Swesnaka Brantwein* (the alcoholic drink of the country) until they absolutely refuse to eat. Out of one hundred and thirty-nine inebriates thus treated by Dr. Schreiber in 1848, one hundred and twenty-eight were cured, four had relapses, seven were brought near to death by the treatment.

The treatment by emitizing alcoholic drinks and by the alcoholizing of all food is sometimes dangerous, and does not contribute, as does homœopathic medication, to the cure of the other vices and failings of the drunkards.

The latter medication is therefore generally preferable to the other two.

X.

NOWADAYS, when people are possessed with the monomania for finding "suggestion" everywhere, one should not be astonished to see allopathic physicians and their patrons explain by suggestion the cures operated by homœopathic treatment generally, and so much the more the cure of drunkenness and other passions brought about by homœopathic remedies. This cure is truly brought about by the remedies and not by suggestion.

1. By means of psychical treatment I usually cure of their passions persons who are treated without knowing it and whom I have never seen.

2. I have made psychical cures which lasted eight years. No cures operated by suggestion have ever been mentioned which lasted so long.

3. Psychical cures are sometimes exceptionally preceded by a drug aggravation, which I should like to be able to spare my

patients, although it is a good sign, and is usually followed by a cure. For instance, a married man, 60 years of age, who had grown more and more jealous during thirty-three years of married life, felt for three weeks, under the influence of a single dose of *Laches*. 200th, a distinct aggravation of his jealousy, of which he was cured in five weeks. This cure lasted until his death—that is to say, eight or nine years.

4. If I were able to cure by suggestion drunkenness and other passions, I should not take so much trouble to seek for the most efficacious remedy in each case, and I should always cure children. Now, quite on the contrary, I cure children of their failings by means of remedies much less often than adults, because remedies are less able to develop reason and sensitiveness to the criticism of those who surround them in children, in whom these sentiments are only in the germinal state, than in adults, who already possess them in a more or less developed condition. Hence, among adults there occurs, under the influence of the remedies administered, an activity of thought and observation which assists the action of these

remedies themselves. Thus I cure of jealousy almost all of the adults, and, up to the present time, I have been unable to cure this failing in children of seven years of age or under.

XI.

THE PHILOSOPHY OF HOMŒOPATHIC DOSES.

DESIRING to explain why I prescribed the most diverse high dilutions for drunkenness, I am obliged to treat of the question of doses in which remedies may be used. In order to solve this question, which divides not only the old and the new schools, but also homœopathic physicians among themselves, I must make use of general considerations, which shall gradually prepare the reader to understand what I am about to set forth.

In the experimental and the observational sciences men have usually, each, a closed field in which they study, observe and experiment, noting indisputable facts of which they hazard the most various interpretations. Unfortunately, as a rule, each individual limits his observations to his own field of investigation, looks constantly through one end of his spy-glass and refuses to look through the other end, by noting in the field of study of each of his neighbors other facts which are equally undeniable. As a result, men of education and learning, having their own minds filled with the facts observed or discovered by themselves, listen only to themselves, will not listen to any one else, and, in that way, become least inclined of all people to acquire new knowledge, and hence most likely to become the slaves of routine.

Prudent physicians, whose duty it is to use for the benefit of their patients all curative doses of the remedies, would act judiciously in imitating, to that end, the eclectic bee, which explores all fields, visits their numberless flowers, compares and judges—since judgment is only comparison—and gathers honey wherever it may. Unfortunately, that is, in the matter of doses, what those physicians do not do who remain fenced within the fields of their experiments, unwilling to see anything outside and therefore unable to judge, since they do not compare the diverse effects of different doses.

Thus allopathic physicians persistently

prescribe remedies only in massive doses, while some homœopathic physicians use only infinitesimal, low, medium or very high dilutions. The exclusiveness of both is often injurious both to the physicians and to their patients. I will explain why.

The remedies prepared by nature or art, like all other matter, present themselves under four conditions—that is to say, in the solid, liquid, gaseous or radiant state. The latter, thus named by the English physicists, Faraday and Crookes, has been called "subtle state" by Aristotle, and "infinitesimal state" by Hahnemann.

According to Faraday and Crookes, when matter is in the solid state its constituent molecules touch and are adherent among themselves. In the liquid state the molecules of matter still touch, but are not adherent. In the gaseous state, molecules of matter are adherent and are more widely separated from all others. In the radiant state the molecules of matter are still more widely separated than they were in the gaseous state.

According to Wm. Crookes, radiant matter constitutes in reality the limit where matter and force seem to shade off into each other.

This makes us understand that under certain conditions, if not under all, the less matter remedies contain the more force they must have. This will be demonstrated to us by the observations which follow.

Paracelsus seems to have had a glimpse or knowledge of similar facts when he describes to us as follows the preparation of his "Arcana," which precede the alkaloids of allopathic physicians and the high dilutions of homœopathic physicians—two preparations with which these "Arcana" have an air of kinship: "Twenty pounds of substance are reduced to one ounce of quintesence, which, however, is the medicinal portion. Wherefore the less matter there is the more medicinal virtues—*Quo minus corporis est, eo magis virtutis in medicinæ*. One thing only is necessary: make Arcana, and direct them against diseases. With them one cures apoplexy, paralysis, lethargy, epilepsy, mania and melancholia—diseases against which the drugs of the apothecaries have proved unavailing."

Observation 1.—An old man in the Charity Hospital of Lyons had for six months, every night, an attack of fever coincident with frequent calls to micturate. I cured this attack with *Natr. mur.* 25th—that is to say, with common table salt in the 25th centesimal dilution. And yet during these six months this old man had swallowed in his victuals a quantity of common salt 100,000 times larger. And, besides, this old man had taken sulphate of quinine and other febrifuge remedies, prescribed in massive doses by a very learned physician, who knew well the resources of allopathic therapeutics.

An objection may be made that a man will not be poisoned, so as to die, by an infinitesimal dose of *Nux vom.*, and will be poisoned by a given ponderable dose of that remedy. That is true. But the same ponderable dose, deadly poison for one person, will be for another, who has great powers of reaction, a remedy that will cure constipation, sick-headache, paralysis. In the latter case, the curative action of this only ponderable dose of *Nux vom.* will often last but a short time, while a single dose of this remedy, in the 30th dilution or the 200th, and more still in the 10,000th, will have a much more prolonged curative action. Thus, for example, this single ponderable dose of *Nux vom.* will be able to cure constipation so as to provoke a few diarrhœic stools during twenty-six or thirty hours, while a single dose of this remedy, in the 10,000th dilution, in one of my patients, treated without his knowledge, provoked similar stools for eleven days in succession, and might have acted still longer if on the eleventh day there had not been administered to him *Veratr.* 3x as an antidote. Even among the high dilutions, the higher they are the more prolonged their action.

For instance, a lady who had an attack of sick-headache every morning was cured for one or two weeks by a single dose of *Nux vom.* 200th, and for six, eight or twelve months by taking another dose of *Nux vom.* 10,000th.

The following facts also demonstrate the prolonged action of high dilutions :

A lady, 28 years old, who had for four years been suffering from acne rosacea, and whose face had, from her infancy, been covered with freckles, took a single dose of *Graph.* 600th, which at the end of five months caused both the acne and freckles to disappear. Would one ponderable dose of *Graph.* have produced a similar effect?

One might consider the curative action of

remedies as a movement communicated to the organism upon a given point and in a given direction. This communicated movement may be brief, like that impressed upon the intestines by purgatives, during from twelve to twenty-four hours, or very prolonged, as in the aforementioned case, by *Graph.* 600th, which took five months to transform the skin of the face of this young lady. The duration and consequently the strength of the movements communicated to the organism by the remedies are proportioned not to the quantity, but to the quality of the movement.

Analogous comparative facts may be observed in other cases of communicated motion. For instance, before the invention of gunpowder the besieged had large machines for throwing stones upon the besiegers, who were thus able to slay their enemies at a distance of one hundred yards at the utmost. Nowadays the besieged, with good rifles, could, with a little bullet and a few grams of gunpowder, kill the besiegers a thousand yards away. It is here again that the duration and the effect of the communicated motion are in proportion not to the mass of the motor, but to its quality. In the same way that different carbines throw the projectile to a distance of from 60 to 1,200 yards, a single dose of the same remedy, differently prepared, prolongs its action during one, two, four, eight, fifteen, twenty, thirty, forty or sixty days.

It seems that the 200th and 10,000th dilutions of the remedy act not only much longer, but also more deeply upon the organism than the third or sixth dilutions of the same remedy. Hence for the lighter, accidentally morbid states one may administer to the sick person diverse remedies in the third or sixth dilution, and then these lower dilutions will not interrupt the long duration of the action of the 200th or 10,000th dilution. And strange as it may seem, the third or sixth dilution of the remedy is sometimes the best antidote to the 200th or 10,000th dilution of the same remedy, which has acted too strongly upon the impressionable organism.

Still one cannot affirm that the curative action of the remedy is always the more efficacious as it is prescribed in the more infinitesimal dose, or in a more radiant state. To so affirm would be to uphold an error that might be very dangerous for the sick.

In many diseases it is better to use remedies not in the 200th or 1000th dilution, but in the third, sixth or twelfth, and at times even in massive or ponderable doses. Thus I do not know that cases of congestive fever have ever been cured with the 200th dilution of sulphate of quinine, but many have been cured by this remedy administered in doses of one or two grams.

I have indeed often prescribed this remedy in larger doses than those given by allopathic physicians. For instance, in certain acute diseases, bronchitis especially, presenting the peculiarity of remittent attacks, growing in gravity and threatening dangerous results, allopathic physicians have slowly succeeded or entirely failed by prescribing from fifty to sixty centigrams of quinine per day during six, eight or ten days in succession. These medium doses, too long repeated, tease, wear out the organism, which then no longer reacts at all, or reacts imperfectly. I have been consulted after these allopathic physicians by the same patients, presenting similar morbid conditions, and I have prescribed quinine in the quantity of one gram, administered in a single dose, each day for three successive days, as if congestive attacks were to take place, and I have cured these remittent attacks and concomitant diseases more rapidly and completely than allopathic physicians had done before in the same person. And yet these physicians had prescribed four or five grams of quinine in eight or ten days, while I only prescribed three grams, but my patient had taken them in three successive days, taking each day one gram in a single dose. It is clear, therefore, that remedies may be prescribed according to diseases and patients in the most varied doses and at different times.

Allopathic physicians unconsciously make use of remedies in the infinitesimal or radiant state—for instance, when they prescribe for their patients the waters of Wildbad (Wurtemberg) and of Gastein (Tyrol). These waters, although they contain no other chemical elements than ordinary drinking waters, cure paralysis. Are not their curative agents remedies in the radiant state, since chemistry cannot discover their presence? Chemistry is likewise unable to reveal the nature of given remedies in medium and high homœopathic dilutions, and yet these dilutions cure many diseases.

The strength of the body seems restored, not only by the remedies in the radiant state, but also by food in the radiant state. This may at least be presumed when we consider the fact noted daily by all men, and thus stated by Professor Rostan: "Food produces this effect almost as soon as it enters into the mouth, or at least as soon as it reaches the stomach. The painful feeling of hunger disappears, to give place to a feeling of general comfort; strength is immediately restored; it seems as if new life were coursing through our entire frame. This effect, however, is not due to assimilation, since not a single nutrient molecule can have been carried into our organs." Thus food, introduced into the stomach and not as yet assimilated, immediately restores the strength. Must this result be attributed to the fact that the food in such a case is absorbed in the radiant state?

Besides, the radiant state seems to manifest itself under other forms also — for instance, under the form of light, heat or electricity. Is light anything else than matter in the radiant state, since spectroscopic analysis enables us to recognize all bodies by means of their respective luminous tints? Electricity, heat and light are not forces, properly speaking, since they cannot be isolated from the bodies which produce them. They are nothing else than these same bodies in their respective radiant states.

It was the odor of matter which gave Aristotle a glimpse of the radiant state which he called *subtle* state, after having noted that one grain of musk, without losing anything from its weight, perfumed for months and months a vast edifice, the air in which was constantly renewed.

Darwin reports a still more astonishing example of the persistence of odor, that modality of the radiant state. "I wrapped," says he, "the hide of a Patagonian deer in a silk handkerchief to carry it home. Now, after having had this pocket handkerchief washed I used it continually. Notwithstanding frequent washings, every time I unfolded it for nineteen months I immediately smelled that odor." This is an astonishing example of the persistency of an odor, which, however, must be very volatile.

The radiant state of matter which, as the preceding facts demonstrate, is produced by nature may also be produced by art. In order to accomplish this, it is only necessary to comply with the direction of the physicists, Faraday and Crookes, who for that purpose recommended that the constituent molecules of each body should be separated so that they should be more distant from each other than they are in the solid, liquid or gaseous state. In this manner, as Crookes says, we reach, I repeat it, "the limit where matter and force shade off into each other;" in other words, there are developed in each body the latent forces which were smothered under the mass of matter. Now that is just what homœopathic pharmacists do when they prepare the infinitesimal doses of each remedy, either by means of successive dilution in a vehicle (distilled water or alcohol), or, if the remedy be insoluble by successive triturations, with sugar of milk.

METHOD OF POTENTIZING REMEDIES.

THE process of dilution most frequently employed is the following, recommended by Hahnemann: To prepare, for instance, the first thirty dilutions of the mother tincture of *Nux vom.* you take thirty vials, numbered 1, 2, 3, 4, etc., up to thirty, and containing ninety-nine drops of distilled water or alcohol. To prepare the first dilution you pour one drop of the mother tincture into the first vial, which you then shake, say, thirty times. To prepare the second dilution you put one drop of the first dilution into the second vial, to which you give the same number of shakes. You continue to prepare in that way each dilution by dropping into each vial one drop of the dilution previously made. Therefore, to prepare the first thirty dilutions of the remedy, there are needed thirty times five grams of distilled water or alcohol; in other words, one hundred and fifty grams of liquid.

To prepare the first thirty dilutions of an insoluble remedy you take five centigrams of the drug, which are triturated with five grams of sugar of milk; in that way the first centesimal trituration is obtained. To prepare the second trituration, five centigrams of the first are triturated with five grams of sugar of milk. The same process is continued up to the third or fourth trituration. The remedies having become soluble can then be prepared by successive dilutions up to the 30th.

The thirty successive dilutions of the remedy constitute thirty different degrees of the radiant state of that remedy. This radiant state has been brought about by separating more and more its constituent particles or molecules from each other. To do this, dilutions and succussions (two factors in all dilutions) have been used. These two factors have the same value, since they accomplish the same end; that is to say, they more widely separate the constituent molecules of any given remedy.

The first thirty dilutions of a remedy have been prepared by employing these two factors. On the one hand, thirty times one hundred drops of liquid; on the other, thirty succussions given to each of the thirty vials;

thirty equal quantities of liquid, multiplied by thirty succussions, give nine hundred as the product.

To a certain extent, one factor may take the place of the other, provided one obtains the same product, nine hundred, to bring about the 30th dilution. When the latter is prepared in this manner it has the same strength as when it is prepared by thirty successive dilutions in thirty different vials. This fact was recognized and this method of preparation was indicated by Hahnemann, who, by one of those intuitions that come to men of genius, had guessed the conditions necessary to bring remedies into the radiant state. After having explained the first process of dynamization with vials, he explains in Section 270 of the *Organon*, in a note to this paragraph, the other process in the following manner: "I have dissolved one grain of *Natr. carb.* in one-half ounce of water mixed with a little alcohol, and for one-half hour shook without stopping the vial two-thirds full, which contained the liquid. I afterward found that this liquid equaled the 30th dilution in strength."

In doing this, Hahnemann may have given

the vial one succussion every two seconds for thirty minutes; in other words, a total of 900 succussions. Now, 900 multiplied by the first quantity of liquid gives as its product 900, which is exactly the same product given in Hahnemann's first process by the thirty quantities of liquid contained in the thirty vials and multiplied by the thirty succussions given to each of these vials; for thirty multiplied by thirty equals 900, and Hahnemann discovered by experiment that the 30th dilution, prepared in either way, has the same strength.

Conforming to the experimental teaching of Hahnemann to separate more and more the constituent molecules of each remedy and bring the latter to a more radiant state, Jenichen substitutes a given number of successive succussions for a given number of dilutions. For instance, to raise Arsenic from the 800th to the 2600th dilution he gives the same vial 51,000 succussions, or about twenty-eight for each intermediate dynamization.

It has been affirmed, without proof, that Jenichen, taking a vial of the fourth centesimal dilution, gave it 1000, or 6000, or 16,000 shakes to make his 1000, 6000, or 16,000th dilution. It matters little, provided that by means of thousands of succussions he has separated the constituent molecules of each remedy so as to bring it into a more and more radiant state and develop its curative powers. Hence it is very justly that the name of potency has been given to the very high dilutions, ranging from 100th to the 40,000th, and that of dynamization to all infinitesimal doses, since this term is more expressive than that of dilution and attenuation. All of this is in conformity with the teaching of Hahnemann, who says:

"The homœpathic remedy in each division or dilution acquires a new degree of potency by means of the succussions which it receives, a means unknown before my day for developing the virtues inherent in medicinal substances, and which is so energetic that latterly experience has compelled me to reduce to two the number of succussions, of which I formerly prescribed ten for each dilution." —*Organon*, § 280.

"The farther a dilution is carried by giving each time two succussions, the more of rapidity and penetration does the medicinal action of the preparation seem to acquire over the vital force of the patient. Its strength is diminished but very little in that way, even when the dilution is carried very far and when, instead of stopping at the 30th, which is almost always sufficient, it is carried up to the 60th, the 150th, the 300th and beyond. Only the duration of the action seems thus to diminish more and more."—*Organon*, § 287.

In the latter paragraph from the *Organon*, edition of 1833, Hahnemann emits two contradictory opinions in affirming that the higher the dilution of the remedy is carried, (1st) the more its strength increases, (2d) that its strength diminishes a little. Later on he confined his practice to the first opinion, experience having led him to give up the ordinary use of dilutions above the 30th and up to the 300th, because he had found the action of these high dilutions too powerful. This is what Dr. Gross, his disciple, tells us in 1846. Hahnemann having but seldom used the high dilutions, had but little opportunity to note that, contrarily to his statement above quoted, the action of the high dilutions is much more prolonged than that of the lower dilutions, as has been demonstrated by comparative experiments.

But as it would take too much time and be too expensive to prepare these thousands of dilutions by Hahnemann's first process, Hahnemann's second process, that of succussion, has been employed instead. By this process, used with exceptional vigor, as related by Dr. Perry in the *Journal of the Welsh Homœopathic Medical Society*, 1851, vol. 2, p. 778, Jenichen prepared the high dilutions of 156 remedies, a list of which was published in said *Journal*.

By means of a third process, utilizing simultaneously dilutions and succussions, a homœopathic pharmacist of Lyons, the late Dr. L. L. Lembert, prepared the high dilutions of 141 remedies, 41 of which were unknown to Jenichen. These 141 remedies were raised up to the 10,000th dilution. Lembert's high dilutions have seemed to me quite as efficacious as Jenichen's.

I advise those physicians who would like to prepare for themselves very high dilutions of remedies, in order to be personally sure of their authenticity, to use Lembert's process, which I am about to describe.

This former professor of chemistry prepared with thirty vials the first thirty centesimal dilutions of the remedies according to Hahnemann's process; then with the thirty dilutions he prepared the high dilutions up to the 10,000th in the manner which I will now detail. Lembert had had manufactured for the preparation of the high dilutions of each remedy a small cylindrical vial of white glass, having the following form and dimensions:

Height of vial, ...	5 centimeters.
Height of the neck of the vial, ...	1 centimeter.
Diameter of the vial, ...	15 millimeters.
Diameter of the neck of the vial, ...	12 millimeters.
Diameter of the opening of the neck of the vial,	1 centimeter.
Lateral orifice placed one centimeter above the bottom of the vial and having a diameter of	6 millimeters.

Into the bottom of this vial, and below the lateral opening, he poured forty drops of the 30th centesimal dilution. Through a siphon connected with a reservoir of distilled water, and placed one centimeter above the neck of the vial, there ran constantly a small stream of water being one or two millimeters in diameter. This thread of water, falling from a height of five centimeters upon the forty drops of the 30th dilution, contained in the bottom of the vial—falling without interruption into the medicated water of the vial—produced incessantly:

1st, dilution of this water; 2d, succussion of this water.

When the water in the vial passed the level of the lateral opening it ran out of the vial.

In order to determine the quantity of water which ran out of the vial in that way, Lembert placed at the distance of twenty centimeters below it a large jar graduated from bottom to top in the following manner:

Knowing that 100 drops, or five grams, of water are necessary to prepare each centesimal dilution, Lembert had calculated that in order to produce twenty dilutions, ranging from the 30th to the 50th, 100 grams of water were necessary. He had therefore poured 100 grams of water in the aforesaid jar and written the number fifty upon the outside of the jar at the upper level of the 100 grams of water poured into the jar.

He thus continued to proceed in the same manner in order to determine what successive levels would be reached in the aforesaid jar by the different quantities of water necessary to prepare the 100th, 200th, 400th, 600th, 1000th, 2000th, 4000th, 6000th and 10,000th dilutions, writing on the outside of the jar the number corresponding to each dilution.

To make the 10,000th dilution he needed 10,000 times five grams of distilled water; that is to say, fifty kilograms or fifty liters of distilled water.

To prepare the 10,000th dilution he allowed the water of the siphon to run for about thirteen hours a day, during from seven to eight days.

In order to get along more rapidly, Lembert prepared simultaneously the high dilutions of six remedies, having, at a distance of forty centimeters, six siphons above six vials with lateral orifices, each one above a graduated jar, such as I have described.

In order to prepare these high dilutions, Lembert thus utilized the two factors ordinarily used; that is to say, dilution in a certain quantity of water or alcohol and succussions. He determined, as has been seen, the exact quantity of the diluting liquid and the approximate number of succussions.* Counting three succussions produced by the distilled water, falling from the siphon into the medi-

---

* These are by no means the exact quantities of the diluting liquid required for the preparation of Hahnemannian potencies (1 : 99); for, practically, the ratio of Lembert's potencies is 1 : 1; however, this would not interfere with their efficacy. B.

cated water of the little vial with lateral orifice, during each second there would have been 1,080 per hour, and 14,040 during the thirteen hours occupied each day for the preparation of these high dilutions; and as it took from seven to eight days for the preparation of the 10,000th dilution, this was brought about by means of from 88,280 to 112,320 succussions; in other words, from eight to eleven succussions for each dilution.

The use of these thousands of succussions, in order to change the molecular state of the remedies and thus bring them into the radiant state—this practice, which at first sight seems, like all new things, so eccentric and ridiculous—is now beginning to be made use of by the chemists themselves, in order to reduce matter to a species of radiant state which favors certain chemical reactions between different bodies. This is related in the following manner, in his opening lecture delivered in 1876 in the medical school, at Montpellier, by the celebrated chemist, Mr. Bechamp, then the dean of that medical faculty and now dean of the Free Medical Faculty of Lille:

"For making alcohol, Mr. Berthelot has

taken the carbonated hydrogen produced by the reduction of carbonic acid. He has caused this gas to be absorbed by means of an ingenious process, which consisted in agitating by a number of succussions sulphuric acid in the presence of mercury. The absorption having taken place, water is added and the whole is then distilled—the distilled product contains alcohol.

". . . I was, in 1856, at the College de France, in Mr. Berthelot's laboratory, when Mitscherlich, the celebrated Berlin chemist and discoverer of isomorphism, dropped in. All at once the following conversation took place between the visitor and the visited:

"Mr. Mitscherlich.—I have tried to repeat your experiment concerning the synthesis of alcohol, but I did not succeed in causing the absorption of the carbonated hydrogen by the sulphuric acid.

"Mr. Berthelot.—How did you go about it?

"Mr. Mitscherlich.—I put the sulphuric acid into a vial with the hydro-carbonic gas, and the absorption did not take place.

"Mr. Berthelot.—You did not put in mercury, or shake the whole together.

"Mr. Mitscherlich.—No.

"Mr. Berthelot.—Then you neglected an essential condition. In order to cause the absorption of thirty liters of bi-carbonated hydrogen by 900 grams of sulphuric acid, in the presence of a few kilograms of mercury, 53,000 succussions are necessary. That is what you neglected to do."

And Mr. Berthelot demonstrated on the spot the reality of the fact to Mr. Mitscherlich.

These 53,000 succussions divide the molecules of mercury and separate them more widely from each other. Then these molecules in their turn divide and more widely separate the molecules of the bi-carbonated hydrogen and of the sulphuric acid, reduce the two latter to the species of radiant state, and permit the sulphuric acid to absorb the bi-carbonated hydrogen. In that case the mercury plays the same role as does the sugar of milk used by homœopathic pharmacists to operate the trituration of remedies and greater and greater separation of their constituent molecules, which brings them into the radiant state and develops their curative powers. Mr. Berthelot, therefore, and all other chemists like him unconsciously make use of this process of succussions which has been used for half a century by Hahnemann and his disciples—a process considered so ridiculous by the ignorant, but so useful, indispensable indeed, by chemists.

This long digression on the subject of the dynamization of remedies seems at first sight to have no connection with the treatment of drunkenness; and yet this digression is necessary in order to justify and explain the use of dilutions in general, and especially of the high potencies, for the cure of certain morbid somatic or psychical conditions, and especially for drunkenness, which is becoming more and more the scourge of families and of modern society. In order to remedy these evils, it is urgent to try the curative means which I propose, since none so efficacious are as yet known.

I am very far, I repeat it, from prescribing exclusively the very high dilutions in my practice, for that would be a mistake that would injure the sick. In many cases the 3d, 6th, 12th and 30th dilutions, and sometimes even remedies in massive doses, are preferable; but in many others the very high potencies are more efficacious, because they have a more energetic, deep and lasting action. I might adduce many facts to prove it. To that end, however, I think it will be sufficient to relate the five following facts:

OBSERVATION I.—Dr. Burnett, professor of materia medica in the Homœopathic Hospital, London, did me the honor of sending to me, in 1882, a gentleman, 34 years of age, who had for four or five years been compelled to abandon the practice of his profession, and during that time had been treated by at least one hundred English homœopathic physicians. He had been declared incurable by two or three homœopathic physicians in Paris. This gentleman came from London to Lyons to consult me. From the 9th of February, 1882, till the 6th of March, 1883, I gave him or sent him, at different intervals, five different remedies, in the 200th, 300th, and 10,000th dilutions. These sufficed to cure him and to permit him to resume the practice of his profession. These five remedies—*Nux vom.* 200th and 10,000th, *Staphis.* 200th and 10,000th, *Calc. carb.* 300th, *Merc. sol.* 200th, *Laches.* 200th —are often used, and doubtless were prescribed by some of the one hundred English physicians who had treated him. But these physicians usually prescribe no higher than the third or sixth dilution to be taken several times a day. These lower dilutions proved inefficacious for five years, while the high dilution just mentioned cured this gentleman completely in fourteen months, as I was informed by Professor Burnett. This fact is very instructive for the homœopathic physicians, who, according to circumstances, would prescribe remedies in all doses and in all dilutions.

When I saw this gentleman taking several times a day the remedy which I had previously prescribed, I quite naturally supposed that he acted in this way in accordance with the advice of his physicians, for in all countries the majority of homœopathic physicians follow this practice. I followed it myself the first twenty years of my practice, because I was surrounded and influenced by *confreres* who had that custom. Since then experience, favorable results becoming more and more numerous, has led me to understand and to accept the teaching which I had received from the celebrated Bœnninghausen in Münster in 1855, and which is the same as that of Hahnemann, who recommends for the cure of chronic diseases to let the indicated remedy, administered in a single dose, act for weeks and even months. (See "Chronic Diseases.") Those physicians who do not conform to his teaching are in danger of meeting with failures in the cases of some of their patients and to see those same patients cured by some more faithful disciple of Hahnemann. Those physicians then demonstrate practically how just is the thought of Dr. Widmann, expressed in the title of his work on "The Sufficiency of Homœopathy and the Insufficiency of Homœopathists," an article published about thirty years ago in two medical journals, one French and the other German. When I do not meet with the desired success in the treatment of a patient, I am often tempted to blame therefor my insufficiency and not the insufficiency of Homœopathy.

OBSERVATION 2.—Mr. X., aged 40, had had a fall from his carriage, which had probably caused a concussion of the spinal cord, for he was no longer able to ride in a carriage, but only in tramways (street cars), which jolt but little, if at all. During eighteen months he was treated without success by three allopathic physicians, two of whom are professors in a medical college, one a hospital surgeon and another a hospital physician.

These three physicians had very probably prescribed for him *Arnica* in ponderable doses, but without result. After those eighteen months of lack of success, Mr. X. having come to consult me, I placed upon his tongue six or seven globules of *Arnica*, in the 200th potency. During the five days following Mr. X. felt a slight aggravation of his lumbar sufferings, after which a complete and final cure of his traumatic pains took place.

OBSERVATION 3.—A lady, aged about 30 years, had the cornea of one eye excoriated by the nail of a child she was suckling. The next year another nursling had again scratched with its nail the cornea of the same eye. For five years this lady felt pain in that eye, and suffered from photophobia, which prevented her working in the evening by the light of a lamp. She had been declared incurable by two physicians, one of whom was connected in a medical school; but she was completely and permanently cured of her traumatic pains by from six to seven globules of *Arnica* 200th which I placed upon her tongue, after having felt a slight aggravation of her pain for five days.

As physicians often have the opportunity of observing similar chronic traumatic pains after a contusion or fall, they will frequently be able to test the rapid action of *Arnica* 200th in such cases, and those physicians will be thenceforth more inclined to convince themselves by experiments that, in other chronic diseases, in which other remedies are indicated, they lose their time when they administer the third or sixth dilution, instead of the 200th dilution of the indicated remedy.

In some acute cases the 200th dilution may cure in less than twelve, twenty-four or forty-eight hours. In proof of this assertion I cite the four following facts, which may be (the fourth especially) tested experimentally by all practitioners.

Observation 4.—A woman, 50 years of age, after an attack of pneumonia, had an attack of acute mania, which was so violent that several persons could hardly keep her in bed, and prevent her throwing herself headlong out of the window. I prescribed for her, to be taken every hour, *Bellad.* 12th during twenty-four hours, then *Stram.* 12th during twenty-four hours, but without success. Then I put upon her tongue six or seven globules of *Bellad.* 200th, which completely dissipated the acute mania in two or three hours.

Observation 5.—A child, 12 years of age, in Paris, suffered from typhoid fever of so ataxic a form that Professor Trousseau, who had been consulted in the case, said to the parents: "I shall not return, for I consider your child as good as dead." Then Jean Paul Tessier, called to treat this so-called dying child, administered in a single dose a few globules of *Arsenic* 200th, and on the next day the ataxic form of typhoid fever had disappeared and had been replaced by the ordinary form of this disease, from which the patient recovered on the twenty-first day, without sequelæ.

OBSERVATION 6.—It is a well-known fact that an attack of pulmonary phthisis often presents several periods of tubercular aggravation, or attacks of suppuration, localized in one or another part of the lungs. By putting upon the tongue of the patient a few globules of *Phosphor.* 200th or 13,000th dilution, at the beginning of each aggravation, I have almost always aborted these attacks in from twelve to twenty-four hours, and if the phthisical person has not become too much worn out and emaciated, he is cured of his disease five times out of ten, but on condition that he shall follow the adipogenous regimen, which will enable him to increase in weight from 100 to 600 grams per day—a result which I have verified in my practice.

At the beginning of these tuberculous attacks I formerly prescribed *Phosphor.* 3d, but it was necessary to repeat the remedy several times a day and for several days in succession, and this third dilution cured much less thoroughly and promptly than the 200th or 13,000th dilution.

One of the ablest homœopathic physicians I have ever known, Charles Dulac, wrote to me on the first of June, 1876:

"Very often a grave affection, which I believed had been cured by the 30th dilution, reappeared at the end of one or two years. Then the 200th or the 600th dilution cured it permanently."

It is often possible to verify the preceding observation, demonstrating that the higher the dilution the more lasting is the cure. I will here complete Charles Dulac's thought by affirming that in some cases the 200th and the 600th are not high enough to produce a permanent cure. To obtain the latter, it is necessary to make use of 1000th, 2000th, 6000th and 16,000th dilutions. For instance, with *Nux vom.* 200th, which had been sent to me by Charles Dulac, I cured a young lady of her sick-headache which reappeared every morning, but then the cure lasted only two or three weeks. I then administered *Nux vom.* 10,000th (prepared by the late Dr. L. L. Lembert), which produced a cure lasting six, eight and twelve months. In other cases I have seen better and more thorough cures following the use of dilutions higher than the 200th and 600th.

But with these facts, to which I might add many others, did not the long digression which precedes the account of them suffice to establish the efficaciousness and sometimes the superiority of the very high potencies, one could utilize for that demonstration a very simple means which I have used for some time with success.

Propose to the skeptics that they shall take daily a single globule of the remedy in the 3000th, 5000th, 10,000th or 16,000th dilution, for several days in succession. Perhaps they will feel no effect the first or second day, but often there will appear on the following days disagreeable, painful, persistent pathogenetic symptoms, which will dissipate their skepticism, and above all will take away from them all desire to try similar experiments again. Certain persons will feel no result whatever from the first or second remedy, but a third or fourth one will produce in them very convincing effects. Then if the skeptics, severely tried by those globules taken daily, accuse you of having put toxic substances into these globules, give them a three hundred drop vial and containing in one hundred drops one of those globules. With this solution, let them, in your presence, make fifteen or thirty successive dilutions, and swallow the one hundred drops of the 30th dilution made by themselves once a day for several days in succession. It is probable that they will experience from these remedies more and more convincing effects—indeed the proofs may be too convincing.

In order to have in these experiments personal certainty, use only remedies proved by yourself and such globules as you will have yourself medicated.

Besides, each day and for several days in succession place one globule upon the tongue of the experimenter. If the latter, I repeat it, feels no effect from the first or second remedy, it is probable that the following ones will make up for that lack of success.

A few boastful skeptics will say that they could take twenty globules at one dose without feeling any effects therefrom. Tell them that they shall take these globules in twenty doses, one per day, and this experiment will probably prevent their being so boastful in the future.

It is very probable that a few persons will be found who cannot be affected by these remedies in high dilutions administered for several successive days. That should not cause any astonishment, since there are exceptional individuals who, naturally or as the result of acquired habit, are unaffected by doses of any given poison that might cause the death of several persons. For instance, certain mountaineers in Styria (Austria) can eat, without harm to themselves, as high as thirty-five centigrams of arsenic. An opium eater at Brousse was able to eat forty centigrams of bichloride of mercury without personal injury. Dr. Pouqueville knew a Turk who had so accustomed himself to corrosive sublimate that he was called Suleymann-yayen (corrosive sublimate eater).

XII.

I ADVISE those physicians who might desire to add, as I have done, to the ordinary treatment of divers diseases the treatment of drunkenness and other passions, to apply this psychical treatment not only to their private patients, but also, and especially, to those who shall visit a free dispensary, established exclusively to that end. These consultants are to return to the dispensary every three weeks, to report to the physician the effects of the remedy.

This psychical treatment in the dispensary presents five advantages not possessed by the practice of that treatment among paying patients.

The first advantage consists in furnishing to the physician the opportunity for a larger number of cures of drunkenness, which, after having benefited the patients, benefit science, and consequently other inebriates. In fact, I cure the drunkards of my dispensary five times oftener than those in my paying practice, and for the following reason: Every three weeks I am given reports of the former, whom I am then able to treat with scientific orderliness and precision and thus increase the chance of success. As to the drunkards of my paying *clientele*, for whom I am consulted at my office, I do not get reports regularly every three weeks, sometimes to lessen the cost of the treatment, but oftener because my patients, so much the more given to reasoning, as they are better educated, reason and reason instead of following with docility the experimental method, as is done by the consultants of my dispensary, under the direction of a physician who is a specialist in this branch. But those well-to-do patrons (among whom I have numbered some who were very wealthy) really believe their experience superior to that of the physician, and therefore begin, leave off, begin again, then again stop the treatment of the inebriates in their families, who, being then less regularly treated, are less rapidly, less often, less completely cured, and often die prematurely from the consequences of alcoholism or licentiousness, its usual accompaniment. It is not, therefore, in the *clientele* of wealthy drunkards that there will be found those fine examples of cures which may benefit science after they shall have benefited the patient first of all.

By contributing to the cure of drunkenness the dispensary has a second advantage, that of preventing the drunkards from provoking discord and misery in their families, to whom they will thenceforth bring their earnings, which had before been consumed in alcoholic drinks.

When these dispensaries shall have become numerous, their third advantage will consist in contributing to the diminution of criminality, which is much increased by alcoholism.

The fourth advantage of such a dispensary is, that it will contribute to the more frequent, extensive and striking popularization of the treatment of drunkenness and other passions. While the paying patients, though manifesting their gratefulness for services rendered, will take the greatest care not to tell their friends and acquaintances that such and such members of their families have been cured of drunkenness or other passions, the patrons of the dispensary will show genuine eagerness to make known such cures not only to their relatives and friends, but also to the people with whom they may converse accidentally for the first time. Their accounts, breathing forth gratefulness, sentiment, sometimes enthusiasm, are repeated by those who listen to them and re-echoed indefinitely by each of the persons who heard them. There is thus made a constantly renewed propaganda of the success of the treatment of drunkenness.

There is in a free dispensary this fifth advantage, that its patients, on account of their personal peculiarities of disposition and culture, are more disposed to accept a new truth, a progress of any sort, than are the majority of paying patients, although the latter are much more intelligent and cultured. It seems to be so for all truths in general.

Before having tested it, one would hardly believe in the practical importance of the following precept of Descartes: "Whenever you wish to acquire new knowledge, erase from your mind all former knowledge."

A child makes an unconscious application of this precept; he does not need to erase what is in his mind, since as yet his mind is a blank. Hence, what constant eagerness he shows in filling it—an eagerness which is kept up by an insatiable curiosity that leads the child to wish to see and especially to try everything. Because of his limited intellectual development he seeks less for intellectual truths than for facts. He has such a desire of assuring himself of the material reality of visible, tangible things, that when, for example, he is shown a statue, he is not satisfied with looking at it, but insists upon touching it and feeling it with his little hands. How eager he is to fill his mind with experimental and observational truths. Therefore, it has been justly said that children look at everything, see everything and wish to try everything. Next to the child, those who are most like him in their almost insatiable desire to see and try everything are those who have little or no intellectual culture. They are not put to the trouble of erasing their previous knowledge, for their minds are nearly vacant, and they are therefore the more eager, like the child, to fill them with the ideas and facts that are presented to them. On the contrary, the more the minds of people are filled with ideas and facts, the less disposed are they to acquire new knowledge, either because they think they have enough, as the result of unconscious pride, or because intellectual weariness, laziness or indifference leads them not to wish to learn anything more. It was probably after having noted this fact that a professor of philosophy in a State university said to me one day: "Educated people are the most given to routine." Two hundred years ago Molière had expressed about the same thought in the following line: "A learned fool is more fool than an ignorant fool."

For the reason which I am about to set forth, cultured people often refuse to acquire new knowledge, even when they might test that knowledge by observation and experiment.

Among learned men, and especially among the members of learned bodies, the majority have gone through a course of philosophy; but too often this philosophy has merely run through their minds, and has left behind not even those elementary principles which are so useful for the guidance of intellectual life: "There are, among others, two kinds of truths—the truths of reason, which are discovered or tested by logic, and the truths of fact, which are discovered or tested by observation and experiment." If a new truth or fact be set forth in the presence of those learned men, the majority immediately want to judge it, to test it by logic, as if it were a truth of reason. They obstinately refuse to test it, to judge of it, as they should, by means of observation and experiment; and sometimes teachers of philosophy, more theoretical than practical, having sometimes a great deal of learning but lacking judgment, would also test and judge by means of logic truths of fact which can only be judged by means of observation and experiment.

XIII.

La Bruyère very wittily describes in the following passage those learned men with narrow mental horizons who, in their supercilious satisfaction with their own special knowledge, will not go beyond the bounds of that knowledge, or see anything outside it, and are therefore thenceforth condemned to intellectual exclusiveness and routine.

"Shall I call him," says he, "an intellectual man who, limited and shut up within some art or other, or even any given science which he practices with great perfection, exhibits outside of that neither judgment, memory, vivacity, good morals nor conduct; who does not understand me, who does not think, who expresses himself badly; for instance, a musician, who, having well-nigh enchanted me with his harmonies, seems to shut himself up in the same case with his lute, or to be, without that instrument, nothing more than a machine out of order, in which something is lacking and from which nothing can any longer be expected?"

* * * *

This class of learned men is so numerous in Europe that, out of a hundred teachers now dead whom I had during my medical study in Lyons, Montpellier, Paris and Vienna, and of whom more than one instructed and charmed me with their special knowledge, I knew but one whose mind was not narrow, and who was not, therefore, a slave to routine; that was Amédée Bonnet, professor of surgical clinics at the Hotel-Dieu of Lyons, and he is also the only one to whose memory a statue has been erected in that same hospital, made illustrious by his teachings. His mind was scientific, literary, artistic, philosophical, and, as a crowning excellence, religious, since the religious spirit, according to the expression of John Mueller, the celebrated historian of Frederick the Great, is "the highest degree of culture, that which completes humanity and humanizes all greatness."

* * * * * *

Unlike the narrow-minded *savants* who have, some of them, remarkable aptitude for mathematics and great contempt for letters and arts, others much talent for letters, but great dislike for science in general, Amédée Bonnet was ready to enter and cultivate all intellectual fields, being convinced that by studying the truths of certain branches of human knowledge one understands better, or even discovers truths belonging to other departments of knowledge. In this way he followed the advice implied in this thought of Pascal: "But the parts of the world are so connected and linked together that I believe it is impossible to know one without the other and without the whole." Hence this eminent clinician was impelled by his insatiable curiosity to desire to study everything within the range of human knowledge; by his *naive* modesty to question, in order to learn, even his inferiors; by his sensitive loyalty to praise the labor of even his adversaries.

Unlike again those *savants* who, innocently believing that they no longer have anything to learn and that they are always right, listen to themselves talk during a discussion instead of listening to their interlocutor, Bonnet listened to the latter with sympathy and curiosity. This surgeon was, to use M. Pasteur's expression, "one of those kindlers of souls, one of those wakeners of ideas, who call forth scientific careers." He was familiarly called the sun of Lyonnese medicine, because he warmed the hearts and enlightened the minds. Hence at the time of his too early demise, at the age of 49 years, there was among the public and the physicians a genuine outburst of regret and admiration which suggested a subscription for the erection of a statue to his memory.

Not satisfied with seeking for truths through his personal labor and in the labors of his associates, Amédée Bonnet sought for it in the practice of physicians without diplomas, as is proved by the two following facts:

By means of the use of glasses of gradually decreasing numbers a man of genius, Henry Schlesinger, of Lissa, in Prussian Poland, had discovered, in about 1830, a means of curing asthenopia, photophobia, presbyopia, myopia, etc. His remarkable cures led the Prussian government to offer him a chair in the faculty of medicine of Berlin, where he might teach his discovery after he should have received the degree of Doctor of Medicine. While he was beginning his studies for that purpose, the Berlin physicians were divided, in reference to his case, into two parties, the progressists, his partisans, and the conservatives, his adversaries. The petty annoyances of the latter compelled Schlesinger to depart, in about 1838, for France, where he practiced his specialty. In 1840 he in vain offered to the members of the Institute and the Academy of Medicine to make known his discovery to them. What respect, indeed, could they have for an oculist who had no diploma? But Bonnet, who above all considered results obtained, requested Schlesinger to practice his specialty in his clinics.

Some time before a professor in a medical college had had himself treated in secret by Schlesinger, who cured him of a chronic affection of the eyes. This professor took the greatest care not to make known to oculists, and especially to his own patients, whom he was treating for similar diseases of the eyes without being able to cure them, but from whom he received fat fees. I learned this at my cost, having been cured by Schlesinger after the professor had failed in my own case. Being informed of this fact Bonnet cried out with indignation, as he shrugged his high and broad shoulders: "I do not understand how one can fail in courage to uphold one's opinion." He might have added, "And sufficient honesty to act, first of all, in the interest of the patients who come to ask us to cure them, no matter by what means."

At another time Bonnet, who had an insatiable love for truth and progress and was no respecter of persons, did better still. He did not fear to lower himself by descending from his chair of clinical surgery to examine the practice of Grenand, a celebrated bonesetter of Lyons. He found there massage, whose application he popularized in regular medicine—that massage with which military surgery cures sprains, they say, three times more rapidly than by means of the old classical medication.

* * * * * *

In France, as in other countries of Europe, law grants the right of treating the sick only to those physicians who have received diplomas from State institutions; and yet, outside of the teaching of the faculties of those institutions, there are many very efficacious methods of medication that are unknown to such faculties. Among others, I shall briefly mention the three following classes of medication:

1st. Homeopathic medication, whose superiority over allopathic medication is demonstrated by its scientific character and by numerous official statistics.

2d. What is popularly called "old women's remedies," and consisting of divers methods used more than a century ago by physicians and forgotten by their successors, but faithfully kept in popular tradition.

3d. Divers medications discovered and used empirically. To this second category of these medications belong, among others, the two following:

A villager who is subject to nephretic colic tells me that when he feels its premonitory symptoms, he gets rid of the renal calculi by drinking a tea made with eight or ten wild-rose berries.

A lady, by administering, morning and evening, an infusion of the dry leaves and flowers of Golden Rod (*Solidago Virga Aurea*) tells me that she cured her husband of an affection of the bladder which had compelled him to use a catheter for a year or more. A friend of homœopathy, not a physician, desired to test the efficaciousness of this plant. He caused the first dilution of its tincture to be taken three times a day by seven patients of from forty-two to seventy-four years of age, who had been obliged to catheterize themselves for weeks, months and years, and cured them so thoroughly that they had no relapses. Surgeons who spend much time and skill in catheterizing such patients for months and years could often cure them much more rapidly by prescribing for them the remedy just mentioned. But they disdain these remedies, proved valuable by popular tradition, and thus make the fortune of the quack who uses them.

* * * * * *

To the third category of these medications belongs the following:

All the vegetable remedies of America, which are being used more and more by the physicians of all schools, were first discovered and used empirically by the Indians of that country.

* * * * * *

XIV.

It will take more or less time, according to the character of the nation where it may be attempted, to cause the adoption of the medical treatment of the passions; and yet it is urgent to remedy the increasing extension of alcoholism among modern nations. Partial success has been met with in those countries in which a certain number of inhabitants voluntarily enroll themselves as members of temperance societies, and pledge to give up the use of alcoholic drinks. But how will you succeed in making temperate the millions of men who are determined to drink such beverages? They either will not, or, as the result of an irresistible impulse, cannot, abstain from them. How, then, can they be given the desire and the strength of will necessary? As I have already said, by administering to them (generally without their knowledge of the fact) remedies whose efficaciousness I have demonstrated and whose differential indications I have pointed out.

* * * * * *

But perhaps the necessity of defending themselves against criminals developed by alcoholism, and of lessening the expenses occasioned to the State by these criminals, will oblige modern nations to encourage the popularizing of the medical treatment of alcoholism.

* * * * * *

Another consideration will show the importance of psychical treatment. The magistrates try and punish criminals; the physicians, who apply with success the medical treatment of alcoholism and other passions, will often be able to prevent the accomplishment of crimes and misdemeanors. If the 180,000 physicians of the civilized world were to use this new medication carefully, the number of criminals would be very greatly decreased. What a beautiful social role they would then play!

* * * * * *

XV.

In 1867 I took advantage of a fortuitous occasion to start a subscription destined to the founding of the homœopathic hospital in Leipsic, the first city where Hahnemann taught his therapeutic reform. Thanks to that subscription, more than three hundred thousand francs have already been collected.

The success of my endeavors in Saxony gave me the opportunity the same year of procuring subscriptions to the amount of 1,000,000 francs for the establishment of a homœopathic hospital in Lyons. If I were able today to dispose of the sums which I raised or caused to be raised I should consecrate them not to the erection of hospitals in which only the lives of isolated individuals can be preserved, but to the founding of dispensaries devoted to the treatment of the passions, especially of alcoholism, the most frequent of all, dispensaries by means of which might be preserved the lives of groups of individuals, families, races, nations. The reader may have become convinced of this as he read the preceding chapters which relate the baneful effects of alcoholism and the happy results of the treatment of this passion. It was after having tested this result that, at an age (61 years) when practicing physicians are usually getting ready to rest, I founded, in 1886, a free dispensary in which I have given, I repeat it, more than two thousand consultations, about two-thirds of which were for sufferers from alcoholism. It is in order to enable all physicians to cure the latter class of cases that I have here published the treatment which has seemed to me most efficacious.

Agreeably to the preceding considerations,

some of the generous donors who found hospitals or endow existing hospitals should consecrate sums of money to the founding of dispensaries. This book demonstrates the urgency of such dispensaries—an urgency which, like the number of crimes and misdemeanors, is growing daily.

INDEX.